SAFER
VACCINES

Perfecting Religious Exemption
from
VACCINATION

STEP UP TO SECURE FREEDOM OF RELIGION

Do not be forced to inject unwanted chemicals

DR. ROBERT CAIRES DC, ESQ.

Became inactive in practice to become very active as a SAFER
vaccines advocate for the CHARITY SAFER Vaccines.

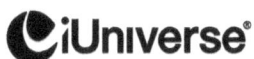

PERFECTING RELIGIOUS EXEMPTION
FROM VACCINATION
STEP UP TO SECURE FREEDOM OF RELIGION

iUniverse books may be ordered through booksellers or by contacting:

iUniverse
1663 Liberty Drive
Bloomington, IN 47403
www.iuniverse.com
1-800-Authors (1-800-288-4677)

ISBN: 978-1-5320-5339-9 (sc)
ISBN: 978-1-5320-5340-5 (e)

Print information available on the last page.

iUniverse rev. date: 01/09/2019

DISCLAIMER

This disclaimer is necessary because I have been threatened to be sued. This disclaimer overrules and supersedes anything written in this book or that is construed from this book. All who read any of the words of this book or learn of this book's contents or recognize its value, merit or benefit or realize it will **stop the AUTISM** epidemic must not do so and **ass**ume it all not true and be not influenced by this book in any way whatsoever. Hopefully this disclaimer will stop me from being sued or attacked.

Everything in this book is not medical or legal advice and chemicals cannot cause injury.

You do not need to be in control of protecting your children, to prevent AUTISM.

Do not read this book without permission from your doctor, lawyer and Indian chief. **I only urge you to not read this book and to not rely on it** for health and AUTISM prevention.

Vaccine Producers do not care more for money than safety; they have no conflict of interest.

THIS BOOK IS a fabrication, a fiction of my imagination and mere opinion; it is devoid of **FACT.**

I do not claim this book's content has merit or
that vaccine chemicals cause AUTISM.

You have no freedom to refuse vaccination or protect your children
from vaccine chemicals. Being enforced to submit children
for unwanted injections is not VACCINATION SLAVERY.

Vaccination mandates are not imperfect law;
do not refuse vaccine chemicalizations.

Give up your liberty if mal-law commands it; you
cannot protect your parental Rights.

You must not disagree to chemically exposing
your children; even if it causes injury.

Parents do not have legal capacity to decide what
is best and/or good for their children.

Parents do not have mental capacity to decide if
chemical injections should not be given.

You need not to reject vaccine injections of anti-
health chemicals; no matter how many.

I do not claim that if you INJECT anti-health
vaccine chemicals AUTISM is likely to occur.

Vaccine Producers' objective is not profiting
by chemicals for profit in vaccines.

Vaccines being chemically safe is as, important
to parents as, it is to Vaccine Producers.

Government mandates vaccinations not
because of drug/vaccine lobbyists.

You must not **disrespect vaccination law,** even if
it secures corporate profit and not health.

Never **question why vaccinations are mandated**
or **if vaccines cause injury or AUTISM.**

Children are not purposely **targeted or programmed**
to take drugs and to be vaccinated.

You must never **think** that **good chemistry equals**
health and bad chemistry equals AUTISM.

Your children can be filled with **vaccine chemicals**
and it **will** not **cause poor health or AUTISM.**

YOU ARE not **A VACCINATION SLAVE** if you
are indentured by law to inject vaccine chemicals.
RIGHTFULLY government, not **PARENTS NEED TO**
CONTROL what is or is not **injected in children.**

Vaccine makers act with impunity when it puts
unnatural to human biology chemicals in vaccines;

WE CANnot CHANGE THIS non-**INSANITY AND**
MUST not **TO SECURE HEALTH FOR CHILDREN.**

You have no **Right of Freedom of Religion.**

You **CANnot Secure Freedom of Religion by Perfecting**
Religious Exemption from Vaccination.

YOU CANnot STRICTLY RELY ON GOD TO KEEP
YOU AND YOUR CHILDREN HEALTHY.

This book was written by a **GHOST** writer, his first name is **HOLY.**

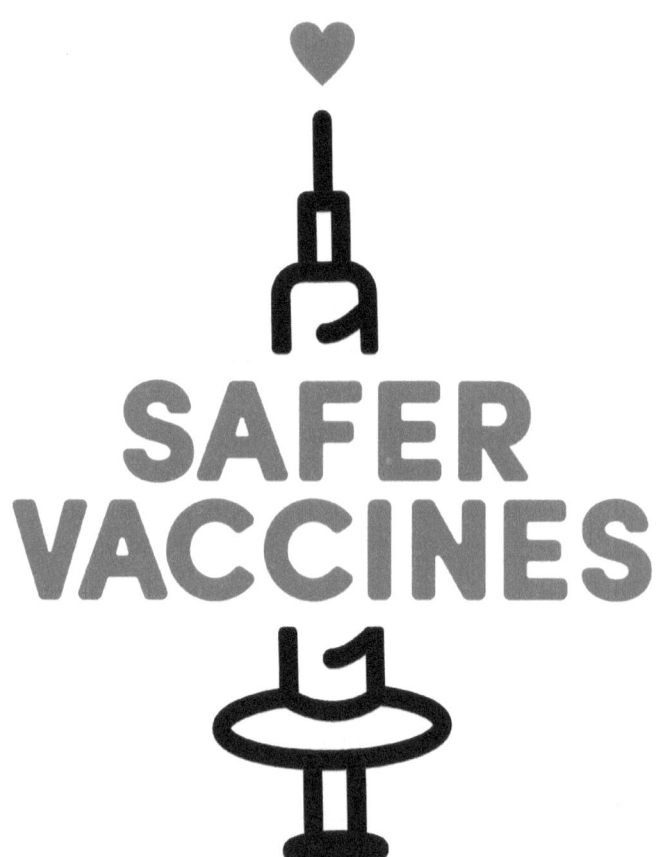

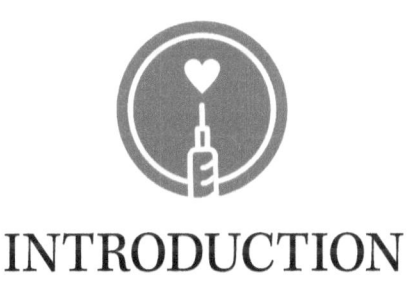

INTRODUCTION

Because politics is intruding upon science and often masters it, medical atrocity is occurring. Vaccines are being injected that are chemically too dangerous to inject. Since, vaccines have become laced with chemicals for profit which are unnatural to human biology, educated and rational people are recognizing its danger and that these tainted vaccinations are an affliction upon health. In addition, many religious people think it a violation against GOD's Law to inject such, alien, unnatural to the body and blood chemicalizations. Manmade law of mandated vaccination is clashing with GOD'S law and that conflicts with the Constitutional protection of Freedom of Religion. There is a feeble attempt to make mandated vaccination Constitutional by sometimes allowing for Religious Exemption from vaccination. Having to obtain a Religious Exemption and the egregious act of questioning one's religion is fraught with impropriety and is not permissive under the Constitution. However, the obtainment of a Religious Exemption from vaccination can save you from violating the vaccination mandate law if you do not vaccinate because of a religious belief that forbids vaccination; it also, saves you from being made to violate your religious conviction not to be vaccinated since, you are exempt from being required to vaccinate due to your religious belief.

The Constitution requires the Free Practice of Religion and thereby, must at minimum afford you the liberty to freely obtain a Religious Exemption and to do so, without being burdened Unfortunately, there are presently many instances when people are drilled with questions about what specifically is their religious belief that forbids vaccination and one's religion is being scrutinized and wrongfully challenged for sincerity. Therefore, it is best to Perfect your Religious Exemption from Vaccination. This book can help you Perfect a Religious Exemption from Vaccination! The book also, covers Autism from Chemicalization and Positive Health Measures. If your religion forbids vaccination or the defiling of your babies' pure biochemistry, this book can help Perfect a Religious Exemption from an unwanted vaccination and/or perfect your Freedom of Religion. GOD has made us in His image therefore, in general we will be healthy if we keep to His perfect design. The Autism epidemic is mainly caused by the injection of unnatural to human biology chemicals found in vaccines; the primary prevention of CHEMICALIZATION AUTISM is the preservation of one's natural and normal biochemistry; keeping with GOD's design.

It is in children's best interest that SAFER vaccines are available. Everyone should be working toward making sure our children are not being chemically compromised with vaccines that contain unnatural to human biology chemicals because it causes abnormal biochemical reactions. Abnormal biochemical reactions equal abnormality and therefore, we must zealously safeguard children from abnormal to the body chemicalizations. SAFER Vaccines, the charity, is dedicated to achieving SAFER vaccines that do not chemically compromise the vital biochemistry or place children in harm's way. Do not be caught up in the idealistic binge of vaccination compliance without tempering it with a good dose of chemical common sense; inject only SAFER vaccines. For the sake of children's welfare, it is imperative that they be afforded SAFER vaccines. To achieve sensible attainable safety results there needs to be anti- vaccine producer's independence when it comes to what chemicals are in vaccines or whether a child is vaccinated and instead, have needed to assure vaccine content safety the requisite parental vaccination determination dependence. To make it much more probable that there are no harmful chemicals in vaccines parents must be FREE to refuse a vaccine they do not deem safe and vaccine producers must be held accountable, responsible and liable for vaccine induced injuries. For the sake of preserving health and fundamental liberty we must perfect Religious Exemption from vaccination. How many babies, infants or children must be injured by unclean vaccines, how many parents must claim their children were caused Autism and how many court cases must find that a vaccine caused yet another precious life an injury until SAFER vaccines become the priority. One should take into account that over a Billion dollars HAS BEEN PAID OUT in an attempt to compensate for the injuries caused by vaccine chemicalization. If vaccines were made SAFER it would not be such, a desecration to blood or human health and therefore, not as sinful or objectionable.

PERFECTING RELIGIOUS EXEMPTION from VACCINATION SECURE FREEDOM OF RELIGION

When mandated healthcare clashes with religion a Religious Exemption from vaccination can save people from either violating the mandated vaccination law or being enforced to violate one's religion. With wisdom, people refuse unsafe vaccinations, based upon philosophy, science and/or Self-preservation. Their stand is to vaccinate only with SAFER vaccines. People do choose not to vaccinate with a too dangerous to inject vaccine and/or a vaccine that is laced with unnatural to human biology chemicals. Parents have a responsibility to secure children's welfare and are executing the parental Right to refuse a vaccine they deem unhealthy; and parents are demanding SAFER vaccines! If you do not understand the laws of chemistry on how unnatural to human biology chemicals cause abnormal biological reactions and thereby, cause abnormality; I strongly urge you to quickly become educated. Know what chemicals are in the vaccine that is scheduled for injection and why unnatural to the body chemicals are objectionable, unwise, unhealthy and must not be injected into tiny babies, little infants and small children. Do not be rendered as, dysfunctional parents by the egregious mandated vaccination law; protect your children always; and in all ways. Those responsible for vaccine content, whom allow unnatural to human biology chemicals

1

in vaccines need to be designated as, dysfunctional, they have lost their moral compass and are bent on making money instead, of children's welfare. It is highly understandable that people have lost blind faith in vaccination and are flocking to rely on their faith in GOD which, is 100% worthy of faith. If you have no faith or trust in vaccines and have faith that GOD will keep your family healthy or that religious belief dictates that you must not inject vaccine chemicalization then, do perfect your Religious Exemption. If I wanted to perfect a Religious Exemption from vaccination, I would use this chapter to assist in doing it!

GOD is the great Enabler! Be FREE to GODIFY your decision about vaccination through Freedom of Religion. If you believe that GOD is on your side that you or your children will remain healthy, despite not being vaccinated; it becomes a reality if your belief is strong. A purpose of becoming more religious, devoting yourself to GOD and raising your level of belief is to channel GOD's power through yourself to do good for yourself and others in GOD's name; GOD is the great Enabler! Injecting vaccination can be an act of being unfaithful to GOD for people whose belief is that GOD enables immunity or keeps one healthy. Thus, to be coerced to vaccinate is to be made to violate one's religion. People must be FREE to live by their religion to allow the Perfect to dwell in the imperfect for we cannot on our own efforts do what is Divine; we need to be FREE to GODIFY; GOD is the great Enabler! There must be liberty to obey GOD's Laws for all your health needs! Freedom of Religion is an inherent Right; no skill is necessary, no sanction from the State is required and it is not an earned privilege. Your religion is between you and GOD! There must be no manmade rules that burden the commandments of GOD. Do you have religious belief that GOD commands you not to defile blood with unnatural to human chemicals?

In religion you may have belief that what you allow into your temple (body) must not cause any harm or spawn abnormal bioreactions otherwise, it violates GOD's Law. What chemicals you inject will either be a stumbling stone or a stepping stone to GOD. There must be liberty to rely upon only GOD to sustain perfect health or for health and not vaccination! Religious Exemption from vaccination assures Liberty to rely upon GOD and not mandated vaccination. We must be FREE to strictly rely upon divine intervention verses mandated medical intervention! The very First Amendment of the Constitution requires that there shall be no law or mandate that directly or indirectly prohibits the FREE Exercise of Religion (FREEDOM OF RELIGION). The First Amendment's religious-liberty clause states that "Congress shall make no law respecting an establishment of religion or prohibiting the free exercise thereof....", this makes enforcing vaccination against your religion illegal and renders it unconstitutional. The ungodliness of injecting unnatural to human biology chemicals is objectionable and violates people's religion. . Whatever you are doing in life, it must make GOD-sense to do it; not nonsense.

If you have a religious belief that your perfectly healthy children must only rely upon GOD to remain healthy and/or that an injection of a vaccine containing unnatural to human biology chemicals defile or makes unclean the sacred body and blood of your children then to coerce, enforce or mandate such, vaccination violates one's FREEDOM OF RELIGION which, is protected under the highest law of the land, the Constitution. Constitutional law trumps State law and therefore, a State vaccination mandate cannot legally require one to violate their religion or religious belief. Mandated vaccination law that does not completely allow for Religious Exemption from vaccination is inconsistent with the Constitution; it violates the Constitution. Even questioning someone's religious belief as, when the State queries for one's religious reason for not being vaccination compliant violates Separation of Church and State. A Religious Exemption can keep you free from sin by not permitting a desecration of your body and blood by vaccination. Relying on vaccination is a sin in certain religions and/or not strictly rely upon GOD or GOD's nature to stay healthy. Do you rely on something much more powerful than mere vaccination; the One who is always pure and trustworthy? You must be FREE to live by GOD's Law!

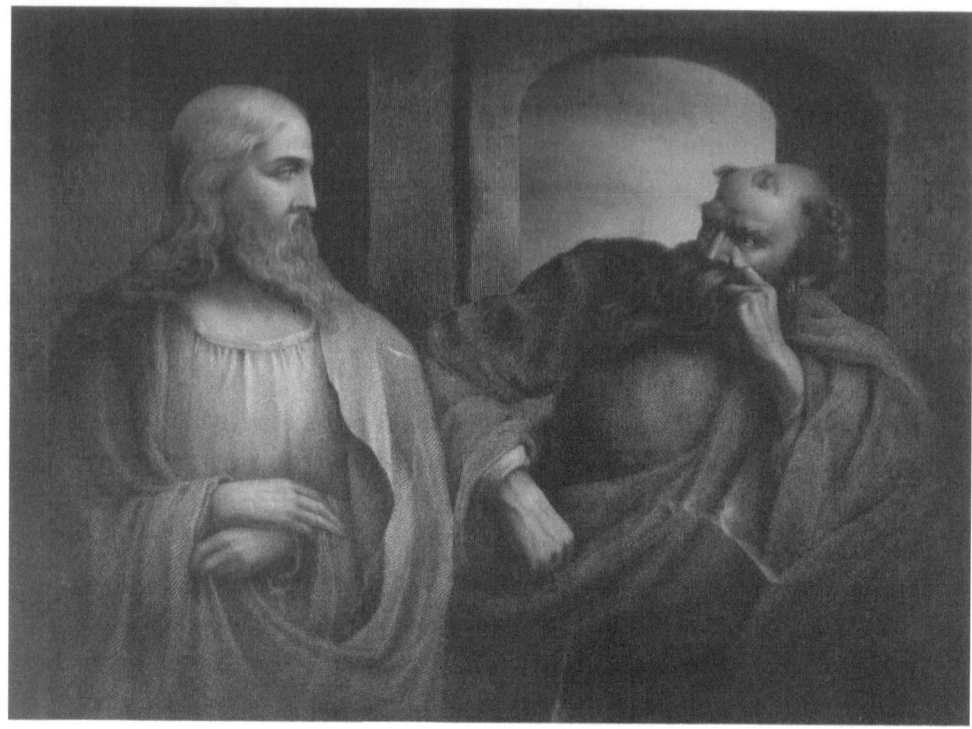

It is unconstitutional to be questioned or judged
about your religion or religious belief.

The level, degree or sincerity of your religious belief cannot, should not and must not be tested or inquired into by government, school boards etc.! You only need to belief that if you pray to GOD for a blessing that it will occur. Whether your faith is strong enough to move mountains or only a single mere grain of sand; it must not be a factor in determining if you can obtain a Religious Exemption from vaccination. People should not be judged on their level of belief or condemned for not having the requisite belief or if it is a sincere belief. Some people believe that they can remain healthy especially, if GOD is asked to help; vaccinations are unneeded for those that have that faith. You can pray for all kinds of things such as, finding your soulmate or the right person to love, getting a good job or even small things in life; certainly, praying for health is a very often occurrence. It is not a question of whether things can occur if you pray; it is a question of how much faith you have or if you believe it can occur with all your heart and if it is GOD's will or part of your divine destiny. Many people who have been sick or even had terminal cancer have become healthy through praying to GOD; certainly, people of faith can stay healthy or even conquer childhood disease with the help of GOD. To enforce vaccination upon such, people may shake their faith, violate their core or cause one to sin. GOD can move mountains into the sea; He created them! The problem is, we are being programmed to need drugs and vaccines, we cannot control our health and GOD has nothing to do with health. Be not deterred, strive to know GOD; throw yourself at His feet!

The concept that everyone must be vaccinated is tribalistic and ritualistic. History has shown that extremism of enforcing medical procedures turns bad and is eventually rejected and is seen for what it really is; the tyrannical mandate of unwanted medical procedure. Today, to enforce inject all with unnatural to human biology chemicalization and make all suffer the consequences of it, is overreaching tyranny. Many, if not most people think that mandated euthanasia sterilization was spawned in Nazi Germany by Hitler but, they would be wrong; it was first spawned here in the United States. In the name of the common good, over 60,000 Americans (mostly children) were enforced to be sterilized against their will and was often done without the victims' knowledge. Finally, it was recognized for the atrocity it is however, it was much too slowly ended. Mandated vaccination is also, perpetrated in the name of the common good; history repeats itself! In the name of the common good sterilization led the way to extermination of undesirables in Germany; it was not that great a leap from the wrong of sterilization to extermination, it was the next level of sick. Today, the madness of extremism has spawned enforced vaccination; children are being assaulted and battered with unwanted injections of vaccines laced with unnatural to human biology chemicals; and injuries are a result. What is next to be enforced upon us in the name of the common good if we continue this path? Mass tonsillectomy has already failed but, I bet enforced genetic engineering will be next; and what will GOD think of that; and will you have to or be able to be Religiously, Exempt?

The chemicals within us dictate our level of health; it is not part of GOD's plan to alter the natural biochemistry with multiple injections of unnatural to human biology chemicalizations. How many unwanted vaccine chemicalization injections must be enforced upon American tiny babies, little infants and small children, without true parental consent or no consent of it or knowledge of it from the vaccine recipient before it is recognized as, being tyrannical medical intervention, self-serving for profit and unjust? When a mandate is locked in by government it becomes a monumental task to end it; it's like moving a mountain; history repeats itself! GOD can move mountains through people whom live in faith! SAFER vaccines may make the enforcement of vaccination a lot less harmful however, the egregious commission of enforcing injections is a harm that can only be rectified by ABOLISHING VACCINATION SLAVERY! Freedom of Religion through Religious Exemption can save you from mandated injection tyranny. Review boards questioning your religion or religious belief often can be cloaked advocates of mandated vaccination in sheep's clothing, having agenda to not grant anyone a deserved Religious Exemption; even if they questioned LORD Jesus, they would not believe a word He says! Best perfect a Religious Exemption and stand strong if they try to make you violate it!

A main reason why people jeopardized life and limb by crossing the vast and treacherous oceans was to escape religious oppression. The initial settlers came to what would become known as, the land of the FREE and BRAVE (America) to seek refuge from the oppression upon one's religious liberty. Our great nation was born out of the need to practice one's religion freely and without persecution or undue influence. How it has come that vaccination has trampled upon Freedom of Religion would be baffling if it were not so obvious that vaccination mandates continue in perpetuity because they turn tremendous profit. Money madness has corrupted the very foundation of America allowing vaccination tyranny to trample Freedom of Religion. If vaccination were not so, unconscionably profitable there would be no vaccination mandates! Mandated vaccinations directly and/or indirectly act as an oppression of religious freedom or do not allow the FREE practice of religion. If your religion dictates that you must not be vaccinated, then no vaccination should be given; religious belief must not be questioned or deemed as, not sincere. The oppression of being mandated to vaccinate and the fact, that vaccine manufacturers act with impunity when it puts unnatural to human biology chemicals in vaccines is tyrannical. We must be perfected in obtaining Religious Exemption and thereby, be secure in our Freedom of Religion.

How one perceives GOD and religion is deeply personal. Intimate knowledge of GOD, recognizing how you personally believe or if how strongly you know the wonder of GOD should not be put to a government test or questioned to see if it fits a set standard which, allows for the golden thread of Religious Exemption. The Free Exercise of your religion must not be sanctioned by government otherwise, it is not the FREE Exercise. Government must not sanction religion! Your religion can instruct you on how to act and/or live and how to protect yourself and your children. You must be Free to consider your body as a temple for the Holy Spirit; part of GOD. The requirement of Separation of Church and State does not allow intimate contact or questioning of one's religion or rendering of any judgment of any kind about your religion. You may be a person whose belief in GOD is not violated by vaccination or has GOD helping at the same time or in tandem with vaccination; that is your freedom. People also, need to be secured in Freedom of Religion to only rely upon GOD, without vaccination!

People can fall in and out of love and what is worse, in and out of their love for GOD and thereby, not adhere to one's religion. Often people develop their own special or personalized religious belief; a religion specific to the individual. People can find religion and/or religious beliefs as, they go through life; it can be contemporaneous with a traumatic life event or be spontaneous as one contemplates vaccination. People must be FREE to ask what GOD would want and follow GOD's will! The duration of one's religious belief is of no business of the State! How long or short the religious belief or how it came about must not be questioned or be a factor in determining religious exemption. In fact, government must not directly or indirectly question one's religious sincerity, it is not the business of government or school boards to determine what or if a religious belief is legitimate or sincere; Separation of Church and State forbids it as, is required by the Constitution. The adage, your body is your temple gives insight that your body or what goes in it, is a matter of religious belief or conviction; what you eat, drink or inject impacts upon one's body religion and/or health. People are religious about health and living in alignment with what they think pleases GOD. The Constitution protects your decisions about health if those decisions are based upon what you think your religion requires. A vaccination mandate must not supersede one's religion or burden the Free Exercise of your religion thus, if you deem your religion forbids vaccination it must not be enforced!

The steering principles that the framers intended to guide or govern the relationship between religion and politics are set forth in Article VI of the Constitution and in the opening 16 words of the First Amendment of the Bill of Rights. The constitutional guarantees of liberty to choose your own religion are what has and still is an essential that makes America great. It is a fundamental principle of democracy that you be allowed to follow what is your religion or your religious beliefs. This all-important principle must be clearly understood, affirmed and vehemently protected by every generation if the American liberty is to endure or be considered rock solid. If mandated vaccinations trample upon religious liberty our American liberty is a sham, a mere experiment gone bad or distorted to the point of being unrecognizable or even opposite of liberty. Vaccination mandates that question a person's chosen religion are an affliction upon our basic liberty and an egregious violation of the Constitution. Do not be coerced by mandated vaccination mal-law to lose your religion; stand strong for your religion! You must be FREE to rely on GOD for health and not be enforced to rely upon vaccination, if your religion so, dictates. Deuteronomy 7:15, "The Lord will keep you free from every disease..." this promises us that if we keep our faith in GOD and do not break our covenant with GOD; there will be no disease or need for vaccination. This scripture is by itself good cause for you to file a Religious Exemption from vaccination if it is your religious belief and in doing so, secure your Freedom of Religion.

Manmade law should not block or deter the Free Exercise of your religion; stand strong against religious oppression!

Because a religion is not looked upon as an established religion or may not fit a chosen definition does not allow for governmental interference in the FREE Exercise of that unique religion. Perfectly, healthy children that have a religious position against vaccination or parents of babies, infants or children of any age that determine a vaccination and/or vaccine injection of a degree of unnatural to human biology chemicals is a strike against one's natural health status and/or is a violation of one's religious belief are having their constitutional guarantee be disenfranchised or violated. Merely, because your belief is unpopular, or practices do not allow for vaccination and/or vaccine chemicalization; you and/or your religion still must be afforded Constitutional protection and Due Process of the Law. Again, if you have a new-found religious belief it must not be questioned otherwise, the requirement of Separation of Church and State is violated. There are over 3,000 religious' groups and there are countless numbers of individuals or families that do not participate in these well-known religions but rather, follow the beat of their very own religious drum, having a personal religious understanding or intrinsic need to please GOD in their own individualized way. The Constitution is clear that government cannot establish one religion over another or selectively advance one religion over another and this anti-establishment of a national or government sanctioned religion or not allowing for deference or preferential treatment of one religion over another poses even more problems for mandated vaccination laws or makes them fatally flawed.

When it comes to health choices or your religious beliefs about what you need to be healthy the road less traveled could make all the difference. Robert Frost wrote, "Two roads diverged in a wood, and I – I took the one less traveled by, and that has made all the difference." Mathew 7:13-14, "Enter through the narrow gate. For wide is the gate and broad is the road that leads to destruction, and many enter through it. But small is the gate and narrow the road that leads to life, and only a few find it." Jesus calls us to travel the road of obedience to GOD's Word = to follow GOD instead of the crowd therefore, if your religion tells you not to vaccinate do not do so; do not follow the crowd of vaccinators. Do not vaccinate because it appears easier, less hassle or that everyone seems to be doing it. When you follow GOD's Law, or the wisdom of GOD is guiding your healthcare decisions, there is a lot less reason to fear the consequences of those choices. John 1624, "Ask and you will receive, that your joy may be full." Always remember that there is nothing in health which lies beyond the reach of prayer except that which lies outside the will of GOD. Your faith can heal you, keep your family safe and healthy; so, live in faith!

Mandated vaccinations that make a feeble attempt at being legal or Constitutional by allowing religious exemptions are fatally flawed because it is the very act of giving exemptions to certain or all religions that have the special need not to be vaccinated treats those people and/or the religion of those people as, sanctioned not to be vaccinated. It categorizes or classifies those with a certain religion or religious belief that forbids vaccination designated as, special entitled to legal dispensation in the form of not having to comply with the vaccination compliance law of mandated vaccinations. All who have the government sanctioned special religious belief are entitled to special treatment in that they do not have to submit to the law to be vaccinated. If you have an approved reason not to be vaccinated based upon a religious belief that forbids vaccination and/or vaccine injected chemicalization then you are singled out for exemption which, is the Establishment or promotion of that religion or religious belief. The legal concept of allowing people to avoid vaccination based upon religion and that for others who do not have that religion or religious belief must be vaccinated creates an unavoidable automatic bias or differential treatment that is based upon religion or religious belief; it is Constitutionally impermissible. Big Pharma and its hordes of lobbyists have thus far, been successful in sweeping this egregious violation of the Constitution under the carpet.

U.S. v. Seeger, 1965, the Supreme Court has asserted the dangers of too narrow a definition of religion by giving conscientious objector status to those who have "a sincere and meaningful belief which occupies in the life of its possessor a place parallel to that filled by the God of those admittedly qualifying for the exemption ...". It is the author of this book strongest opinion that the requirement of "a sincere and meaningful belief... goes way beyond what is constitutional; the act of religious sincerity goes to far and brings government into the seat of religion or causes government to make religious determinations that are way outside of Separation of Church and State requirements. In a mandated vaccination or vaccination compliance query the foundation of government's authority or a school board to inquire about someone's objection to be vaccinated based upon religion or religious belief to determine if it is sincere is based upon the above Supreme Court case. How on earth or rather, in heavens name can someone determine if an individuals' religion or religious belief is sincere; it is a total bogus attempt at being all knowing. Be FREE TO REJECT INJECTIONS based upon religious liberty; it is A MATTER OF SUPREME LIBERTY!

Religious Freedom is under attack and if we do not protect this most essential liberty it will be lost. Blood in many religions is considered sacred; certainly, people are religious about what flows through their vital bloodstream. FREEDOM to prevent an injection of unnatural to human biology chemicals into one's body and blood is part of more and more people's religion. The bill, NY A1810 (17R), from Assemblyman Jeffrey Dinowitz (D-Bronx) and state Sen. Brad Hoylman (D-Manhattan) to eliminate the religious exemption entirely never made it out of committee. The bill, NY S2955 (17R), that would have required school districts to report the number of religious exemption requests received and accepted also, failed to make it out of the Senate Education Committee. The deep pockets of Big Pharma and its droves of lobbyists will not cease in seeing to it Religious Exemption from vaccination does not prevent increased profits from enforced vaccination. Families that seek religious exemption are put through the 3rd degree. Schools acting as judges in determining what is a valid religion or not is crazy and egregiously unconstitutional. It is unamerican that a government employee or school committee, panel or board can be empowered to tell a parent what that parent's religion teaches or that the parents' a religious belief is a sham, invalid or not sincere. Indeed, people came to what became America to escape this kind of persecution upon one's chosen religion. It is totally disconnected to Freedom of Religion to be denied a religious exemption or to be overburdened to answer questions about one's religious beliefs.

States that unconstitutionally have no religious exemption or are in a State that commonly refuses or invalidates religious exemption are making people leave that oppressive State just as our forefathers or ancestors found they had to leave other countries to come to America to freely practice their chosen religion. When vaccination mandates cause people to not travel freely from one state to another it is yet another violation of the Constitution. In the above paragraph people were caused to leave a State in order, to freely exercise their religion and/or not be vaccinated and that is a violation. When someone is caused either directly or indirectly to not to enter or live in a State because that of that State's mandated vaccination law and/or that they are not free to live by their religion or not enabled to have a religious exemption from vaccination that is one's liberty to travel freely between the States.

How long can you remain unvaccinated in the State that requires vaccination before you are considered breaking the law of that mandated vaccination State; is a question that indicates how unworkable and unconstitutional mandated vaccination law is. Not all States agree about religious exemptions and that makes mandated vaccination without religious exemption and/or without philosophical exemption or easily obtainable medical exemption a legal mess that points to only one conclusion and that is mandated vaccination is illegal especially, if it does not allow for completely easily obtainable and/or unburdened exemptions. Imagine innocently entering a State that requires you to be vaccination compliant and you and/or your children are not vaccinated either because of your religion or philosophy or health issues that the State your presently in does not agree with? They will chase your children down with a huge vaccination needle particularly if they go to daycare and especially, if they go to public school. If the reasonable person would feel that they had to leave that State, then the reason that caused the family or person to leave is unconstitutional (that being the State mandated vaccination law).

The degree of egregious violation imposed by mandating vaccination despite it violating one's religion or religious belief is of the highest magnitude of violation against Freedom of Religion. Forgive my humor on such, a serious topic in depicting how much more egregious injecting a child with a vaccine chemicalization is when the religion of the parents and child forbid it. Envision a lobbyist for Budweiser beer asking for a meeting with the Pope to make a million-dollar donation and the lobbyist requires that before Budweiser commits to donating the million that the prayer having the words my "daily bread be changed to my daily bud". A Cardinal after speaking with the Pope says, "my son this is a prayer that is said by millions of people around the world, I am afraid what you ask for is impossible however, we would love the donation". The lobbyist then states, "my last and final offer, Budweiser Beer will donate the huge sum of 100 million. The Pope finally speaks and commands to his Cardinal, "get that contract out with Wonder Bread." This little humorous scenario depicts how lobbyists with big bags of money are ruining the world as we know it. Nothing is sacred, they will seek to alter or manipulate anything that can benefit their self-serving agenda even if it means mandating vaccinations against people's will or if it is against one's religion. Money madness is taking over as, our freedoms are being violated in every which way.

Compare the levels of violation against Religious Freedom in the following scenarios. What is a greater violation when someone is not permitted to dress according their religion or when one is enforced to inject their children with a vaccine chemicalization that is not only has unnatural to human biology chemicals but has been known to cause signs, symptoms and/or injuries and is not in accordance with one's religion? What is more of an egregious violation against person or religious liberty to be required to work on Sunday that is designated as, the day of rest according to one's religion or be vaccinated against one's religion. What is a worse violation against the FREE practice of religion to be disallowed to eat the bread of life or swallowing the wine that re[resents GOD's blood at church because it is decreed by government that such, community distribution is an unsafe practice, having too great of possibility of spreading communicable disease as, compared to being enforced to be stuck with a needle and injected with vaccine chemicalizaton that is known to cause harm and is against one's religion or one's religious belief that you should inject such unnatural to the body chemicals into sacred blood and/or rely on man instead of GOD to remain perfectly healthy. The degree of violation against Freedom of religion is not even comparable; the enforcing of perfectly healthy babies, infants or children to suffer an unwanted vaccine chemicalization by injection that is not permitted according to one's religion or religious belief is off the scale of comparison and ultimately much more egregious against the FREE Practice of Religion. Mandated vaccination is a most egregious violation when imposed or forced upon someone especially, when it goes against one's religion. People whom have been violated with an unwanted vaccine chemicalization that have a religious conviction against it, must both deal with the consequences of the negative to health chemicalization and live with the sin of such, chemicalization that violated one's religion.

Religious liberty has been called America's "first liberty" because freedom of the mind is philosophically and logically come prior to all other freedoms protected by the Constitution. The power of the State or laws must not impinge upon one's Freedom of Religion. Religious liberty is a natural or inalienable Right that must always be beyond the reach or power of the State to override, sanction, deter, remove or confer. The act of government or sanctioning a school board to question one's religious belief is coercion and control over one's religion or how you interpret your religion. There are really 4 kinds of exemptions: the medical exemption (a health issue), the philosophical exemption (it is not rational to vaccinate, or you think it too dangerous), the serological exemption (you prove your child already had the disease naturally) and the all-important religious exemption (that is protected under the Constitution as part of Religious Freedom). Do not lose your religion or be made to deny your religion or compromise your religious belief; stand strong against vaccination if it suppresses the Free Exercise of religion!

The First Amendment's religious-liberty clause states that "Congress shall make no law respecting an establishment of religion or prohibiting the free exercise thereof....", this ensures that religious belief or non-belief remains voluntary, FREE from government intrusion or coercion; it renders enforcement of the inferior mandated vaccination law as, unenforceable and as, unconstitutional when it attempts to enforce vaccination or question you when you fill out a religious exemption form or merely state you have a religious exemption that vaccination is against your religion. GOD knows the workings of the body, there is no greater expert on biology or what chemicals the body needs to be healthy and what chemicals are bad for you. The neurobiological, mental and SPITUAL adverse effects and/or trauma of being enforced to inject unwanted vaccinations which, have unnatural to human biology chemicals that is against your religion to do so, only GOD totally knows.

The Free Practice of Religion is substantially burdened by mandated vaccination laws that dictate, control or question religious convictions. The history of our country has gone from mere toleration of religion to FREE exercise; there is no valid legal ability to question someone's religion authenticity or sincerity. Religious exemption from vaccination must be respected and unquestioned. Perfectly healthy unvaccinated children are perfectly healthy with no current health issue therefore, they are no threat to others. The only real threat is from vaccine chemicalizations that have unnatural to human biology chemicals; the so called, vaccination court has proven that by awarding over a billion-dollars to those proven injured by vaccinations. Freedom from unwanted vaccine chemicalization is required to achieve and keep SAFER vaccines and Religious Exemption from vaccination is required to maintain the highest law of the land.

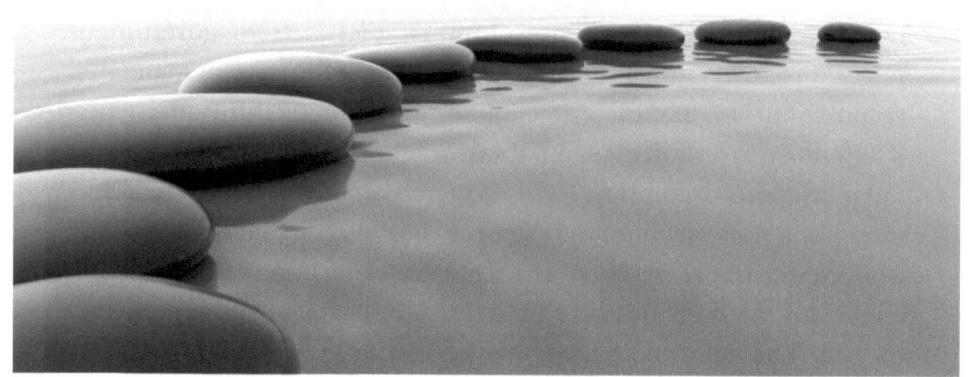

Perfecting Religious Exemption is the necessary
stepping stones to Secure Freedom of Religion.

Perfectly healthy children pose no real threat to others; it is mere
conjecture that they may pose a threat and law must not be based upon
a non-threat or fiction of a threat or mere conjecture of it therefore,
there is NO COMPELLING REASON, nor rational to deter
religious belief or overpower one's religious conviction or disembowel
a religion that is not consistent with mandated vaccinations. If you
have long-term religious beliefs or have a sudden epiphany or great
awakening and thereby, develop brand new religious beliefs; you
are protected under the Constitution to live by all your religious
beliefs without governmental intrusion, coercion, condemnation;
no law should supersede your religious beliefs. The Constitution is
under attack when religious exemptions are attacked thus, religious
exemptions must be zealously safeguarded. Your religion may call
upon you to protect your children from chemicalization harm.

One should not be scrutinized for their religious beliefs and/or
be made to be tested about them thus, NO religious testing! Your
GOD and/or religion is for only you to interpret and decide if your
religious beliefs or convictions is a matter of utmost privacy or to be
broadcasted; at no point can government burden you or conflict you
about your religion or cause you either directly or indirectly to reveal,

test or put on trial your Religion or Religious beliefs. FREEDOM OF RELIGION and Religious Exemption from vaccination is A MATTER OF SUPREM LIBERTY especially, when parents are securing their perfectly healthy children in the protection of their faith, religious belief or conviction and/or religion! Our Constitution recognizes GOD'S LAW and the FREE exercise of religion to satisfy your GOD'S LAW.

You must be FREE to solely be resistant to disease by your natural built in immune system and if it is not powerful enough; be FREE to solely rely upon all-powerful GOD. I may not be powerful enough, but GOD is on my side and is ALL-POWERFUL. Someday soon, if we do not zealously protect the Free Exercise of Religion, government under the direction of lobbyist seeking to obtain profit for the corporation it represents, will achieve egregious affliction against our bodies and Freedom of Religion; it will likely come in the form of other mandated medical intervention such as, but not limited to, mandated stem cell and mandated genetic engineering. Insurance companies will try to deny issuing policies if you are not genetically modified or compliant will the latest cutting-edge science breakthroughs for health except; it will cut into people's religion and violate individual's religious beliefs or convictions if they are made by mandate. To succumb to whatever, future healthcare may come of age and be suggested for mandate when it crosses over into the religious realm and/or violates one's religion is a future that must guarded against and by correcting the obvious violation of people's religious beliefs from mandated vaccination is a necessary step to protect to stop the injustice of today and to protect our future. No healthcare should be mandated especially, when it is against one's religion. No one should be molested, assaulted and battered into unwanted medical intervention when they are perfectly healthy in no current need of the medical intervention for to do so, is like or worse than being raped. No one should be forced, enforced or coerced into anything that they consider evil or that is deemed by the individual as against their religion or GOD's divine law! However, let me be clear, I am for vaccination, I am for SAFER vaccines that are administered to those who do not have a religious objection and/or other objection.

If science produces a viable way to prevent cancer by genetic engineering or other means that would be fantastic however, to enforce it upon FREE people and/or to make people whose religion does not allow for it must not be allowed and must be considered unconstitutional and unamerican. The mandated vaccination laws are the first cut into Parental Liberty, Right to Self-determined Healthcare and Freedom of Religion; and the first cut is the deepest. The goal is not to suppress science and to be FREE to benefit from it however, not oppress Rights or impinge upon the Free Exercise of one's Religion. We can have a bright future but, we must tread carefully and correct any hint or actual affliction upon Freedom of Religion. Law must never separate People form their GOD! Perhaps, Freedom of Religion is protecting us from catastrophic man-made epidemics. In Psalm 46, GOD says," Be still and know that I am GOD." The Hebrew word for "still" means to "cease striving" which can mean to those whom have the belief that when it comes to considering preventative healthcare or when in the midst of trouble or a health issue "be still" and trust in GOD; do not seek vaccine chemicaliztion by injection, know that GOD is your refuge and strength and that you can rest in GOD's care.

Oppression of religious liberty or of one's personal religious belief has been curtailed as time progressed however, mandated vaccination without religious exemption is a giant step back in time as, it is an unacceptable oppression of religious liberty, an anti-free exercise of religion. History shows that individuals who first had a new interpretation of the Bible were put to death for doing so. The first English version of the scriptures made by a direct translation from the original Hebrew and Greek, and the first to be printed, was produced by the hand of William Tyndale. He was not only met with coercion and bitter opposition for his so called "untrue translation" he was publicly executed and burnt at the stake in October 1536. As usual authority got it wrong in that many later in time Bibles were based upon Tyndale's translation. Tyndale's personal understanding became the foundation of many subsequent versions such as, the Coverdale, 1535; the Great Bible, 1539; the Geneva Bible, 1560; and the Bishops Bible, 1582 and others. The King James Version considered all of the above Bibles so, Tyndale's was put to death, but his work on Religion or interpretation of the Bible lives on to some degree. No version of the Bible and no religion is perfect. We have come a long way from once putting people to death, if we do not agree with their religious ideology or personal beliefs, to now, questioning people's Religious Exemptions; it is still oppression and it is against the Constitution requirement of Freedom of Religion. Your relationship with GOD or what is the religious rules of your personal religion is for only you to decide; it certainly is not for government or a government sanctioned school board to question or condemn or determine if sincere. It makes no difference of your religion is popular religion or not, the constitution protects your Free Exercise. Today no one is put to death for their unique religious belief however, you can be subjected to an inquisition about your religion or religious beliefs and that must be declared illegal. Nothing detrimental such as, suffering your children with an unwanted vaccine injection should be permitted especially, if it is against your religious belief or your religion forbids vaccination.

Since, the sacred ground of what GOD dictates to you is now being tread upon by government intrusion and commonly challenged by those who benefit from enforcement of vaccinations with no realistic religious exemptions, it is wise to be best prepared for such, attack against your religious liberty. There mal-intent is to ask you blatantly invasive illegal questions or quasi legal questions about your religion or religious belief which, requires you not to submit to vaccination in an effort to put your religion to the TEST or rather, put you to the TEST to see if you truly have a requisite belief that will sanction a government approved religious exemption from the mandated vaccination law. What you state will be held against you in order, to deny your exemption and enforce vaccination. Hope for a fair and unbiased assessment without prejudice.

They may attempt to show that you do not have what it takes to allow for a religious exemption. They may designate your belief as not a "sincere" religious belief or conviction or that your reason not to vaccinate is not material to your religion or it is not a bonified or all-important part of your religion. Nobody but you can determine such a thing; only, you know how you truly feel and think about your religion or religious belief in just how vaccine chemicalization injections violate GOD's divine law. It is an overburden and at times impossible to have to prove to total strangers whom perform the inquisition which, you must go before that you have religion or that your religious conviction against vaccination is sincere (real). In a total violation of Due Process, a school board acts as judge and jury in determining if your Constitutionally protected Freedom of Religion allows whether you will be permitted a Religious Exemption from vaccination. Best Perfect Religious Exemption from vaccination by documenting what scripture you live by that you interpret is violated if you or your children are made to undergo vaccine chemicalization. Make it abundantly clear that your religion dictates you to rely upon GOD and His nature for health and/or how vaccination is a breach in your faith and/or that it is not in GOD's plan for you.

Besides stating emphatically or with extreme emotion that is one could take steps to show it is. Husband and wife before having children could write up a religious belief document about why their chosen religion prevents one from being vaccinated and then when you have children it could be used as factual proof of your religious belief and that it has been long held and that it was so, important that it was written as law of your religion to live by even long before you had children. Mailing it several times to yourself and not opening it may be a way to memorialize your long-held belief that equals sincere or genuine religious belief. The post mark on the unopened envelope is collateral or supports how long you have had your anti-vaccination religious belief. Perhaps the dramatic opening of the letter in front or witnessed by those inquiring minds serves as proof of your sincerity of your religious belief and can be enough to win your cause and end the invasion of privacy and attack on your Freedom of Religion. Of course, what is in the letter is all-important! They may have it wrong that the longer you have a belief the sincerer it is. It is not how long held your belief is or how much faith you have; it is a matter of how powerful GOD is!

The words that are in the letter should make it clear why you cannot submit to vaccinations and/or state clearly what your religious conviction is and how it does not allow for vaccination. For example a growing religion has a religious faith or belief that if we are born perfectly healthy we should remain healthy and rely strictly upon prayer and GOD to do so and/or that the voluntary or non-voluntary piercing of skin violates one's body and GOD and/or the injection of a vaccine that contains unnatural to the contents or unnatural to human biology chemicals violates one's body according to your religious belief and/or violates GOD's law and therefore, would be a sin. The belief that GOD will provide for you and that GOD protects you and that you must only rely upon GOD and his nature for health make submitting to a vaccination forbidden. According to your religion the injection of a vaccine defiles your sacred blood. If you break GOD's law and submit to vaccination you may go to hell and may fall from the grace of GOD in perfect health to be befallen in sickness due to not following what you know to be GOD's will. Your body is your temple for the Holy Spirit and not for man-made vaccine concoctions that claim to be good for you. Vaccination reliance hysteria may be considered a religion but, not yours!

They may be so bold to ask, have you heard that vaccine safety is controversial or can cause Autism to try to avert your religious belief from why you do not allow vaccination to a philosophical reason or one based on science or so-called unproven science or based on irrational fear. If you say yes, it could be construed that your religious belief is a sham and the real reason is your fear of vaccination. It is possible to have a sincere religious belief and have a philosophical reason or intelligent understanding that vaccinations are causing injuries however, the reason you are there is to speak to your religious reason not to be vaccinated and any other inquire is irrelevant to the issue before the board of inquiry. Once you open the door to the conversation about anything other than your religious exemption someone may get it wrong or seek to wrong you and not approve your meritorious religious exemption and/or your belief as valid or sincere. Stick to why GOD wants you to follow His Word and not defile your baby's blood.

Many vaccines violate one's religion because the vaccine production utilizes aborted fetus tissue. Do your own research and have the facts to help assure your religious exemption. Vaccines such as, Polio, Dtap/Polio/HiB Combo, Adenovirus, Hep A, Hep A/Hep B Combo, MMR, MMRV Pro Quad, Rabies, Varicella, Shingles vaccines, HIV, influenza and tuberculosis vaccines have been found to contain DNA, cells, cellular debris and protein from aborted fetus tissue. The list of vaccines that may violate your religion is longer and keeps growing so, do your own research. It might aid your goal of a religious exemption by stating that the Pontifical Academy for Life strongly condemns the development of vaccines from fetal tissues if it coincides with your religion. Also, the fact, that religion is violated because the act of injecting or consuming such, aborted fetus containing tissue makes one a cannibal; the amount of human tissue consumed does not refute the fact that it is a cannibalistic act to inject or swallow such, vaccines.

If you want to further your position you can bring a Bible or recite scripture that supports, your religious conviction or interpretation and/or the use of aborted (killed) babies. Psalm 22:10-11; & Galatians 1:15), are blessings from God (Genesis 1:28; Genesis 4:1; and Psalms 127:3 and 113:7-9), are valued and loved (Matthew 18:1-14 and 19:13-15), are created in His image (Genesis 1:27), and their killing is condemned (Psalm 106:35, 37-38). The prophet Amos condemns the Ammonites because they "ripped open expectant mothers in Gilead" (Amos 1:13) and child killing was one of the major reasons that God's anger burned against the Kingdom of Israel bringing about their destruction and exile (2 Kings 17:17-18). However, you may have created a new religion that does not use any Bible or had a dream that inspired your religion that makes vaccines that use aborted baby tissue a violation of your new founded religion.

Your religion may require you to keep your blood and your children's blood pure. Blood is considered sacred in many religions and it is in the Bible (Leviticus 17:10, Leviticus 17:11, 17:14, Deuteronomy 12:23, Acts 15:20, Genesis 9:4 and Acts 15:29). Therefore, to inject your baby or baby's blood with a vaccine that contains unnatural to human biology chemicals defiles the blood. In addition, vaccines contain biological agents or use materials of biological origin and can be contaminated with microorganisms. The use of a school committee that is sanctioned to seek to destroy religious exemptions subverts Freedom of Religion and directly violates the Constitution. One should not have to recite scripture to bolster one's religious belief; one should merely have to state that they have the religious belief such as, keeping blood pure and/or sacred is necessary according to one's religion and that vaccine chemicalization makes blood impure. GOD and/or religion sometimes defies logic and cannot be proven and that is what faith is all about. Government or its sanctioned empowered school panel cannot determine if someone's faith is legitimate, logical, makes sense, sincere or truly held. The highest court of the land, the Supreme Court needs to end this charade and end the affliction upon the First Amendment by securing Freedom of Religion and/or Religious Exemptions.

Depravation of one's Freedom of Religion is a most serious offence and depriving an individual of their Religious Exemption from vaccination is a depravation of Free Exercise of one's religion and is repugnant to the Constitution; a most egregious violation of the Constitution. School boards have an inherent conflict of interest in accessing or determining if you have a valid religious exemption because it benefits from denying your religious exemption. The school or school district can lose its federal funding if its vaccination compliance level falls below a certain level therefore, the select panel or school board has a bias or preconceived agenda to deprive you of your bonified religious exemption. If you determine that you have been a victim of such, bias or prejudiced because of your belief you could consider litigating against the board members in their personal capacity for it. If a board member acted with obvious bias, mal-intent or acted negligently the depravation of your Freedom of Religion by denying your Religious Exemption takes on the additional cause of action. People who find themselves faced with this deprivation or being commanded to violate their religion are placed in an untenable position and may be forced to be civilly disobedient but, it is at no fault of their own. The inquisition into one's religion or religious belief is wholly unconstitutional and reeks of impropriety. No one has legal capacity to be judge and jury over your religion or supersede what you have deemed your religious belief; to do so is a gross injustice! Stand firm in the truth of what you know is GOD's Word, remain pure and holy.

Psalm 27:7-14, When You said, "Seek My face," my heart said to You, "Your face, Lord, I will seek." v.8, when faced with adversity or the dilemma of vaccination or those that want to enforce inject a vaccine chemicalization your Freedom of Religion allows you to run to GOD and have sanctuary in GOD from being defiled by injection. If your religious belief is that it is against the will of GOD to inject into your baby or child unnatural to human biology chemicals and/or that vaccines manipulate or cause your body to react or forces a manmade or medical intervention induced biological reaction, then that religious belief or religion must be respected. It is quite possible that you may also, have what may be viewed as, a consistent or inconsistent philosophy or intelligent procured understanding that to inject such, vaccine chemicalizaton is unhealthy or too dangerous. The fact that you have both a religious conviction and an understanding that it is unhealthy to inject a vaccine chemicalization does not diminish, disembowel or transgress your religious exemption or can be considered a factor in determining if religious belief is sincere. Inconsistent statements or consistent statements about the science of vaccination or how it violates you may be considered irrelevant to the acceptance of your valid religious exemption.

It is not as if vaccination mandate is only about protecting us from harm after all, vaccination is big business and Big Pharma is extremely active to assure vaccination is mandated in perpetuity. If there was no money to be made from mandated vaccinations, then vaccinations would not be mandated; it more about money than the safe keeping of our children. There are chemicals in vaccines that are chemicals for profit and not safety. Timothy 6:6-10, "The love of money is the root of all evil, for which some have strayed from the faith in their greediness." V. 10. Many have lost their morale compass in mandating vaccination and the amount of money spent to program the population into robotically vaccinate and the hordes of lobbyists with their mega-bags of money to mandate more and more vaccines to make more unconscionable profiteering evidences that evil is at work. The YOUR CHILD, YOUR DECISION initiative of the charity SAFER vaccines that seeks to correct the unconstitutionality of mandated vaccinations and the liberation of one's Free Exercise of Religion by assuring absolute liberty to Religious Exemption. Money making must not overcome parental protection of children or be permitted to have your religion or religious beliefs questioned or be approved of.

Referring to the Bible or what JESUS or GOD said to support your religious conviction against relying upon vaccination is a most powerful. Isaiah 40:29-31: "He gives power to the weak, and to those who have no might He increases strength…" Here it is revealed that if you rely on the LORD you will have omnipotent power to be healthy whereas, if you are infatuated with man-made medical intervention such as, vaccine chemicalization injections you may feel powerless. If you are FREE to practice your religion, to solely rely upon your belief in spiritual power you will be strengthen inwardly by GOD's omnipotent power. The power of the Holy Spirit is the same power that "GOD raised Christ from the dead" (Ephesians 1:19-20, NIV) and is the power that you long to rely upon instead, of mandated vaccinations. Instead, of being a robot and just being vaccinated because you are told to or being enslaved to vaccinate due to an erroneous mandated vaccination law you are FREE TO BE EMPOWERED BY THE LORD JESUS by allowing LORD JESUS to walk around in your body and live His resurrection life in and through you. As GOD wills, it will be done, Mathew 8:27, "So the men marveled, saying, 'Who can this be, that even the winds and the sea obey Him?'" You must be FREE to seek the power of GOD for your health needs and not be broken by a mandated vaccination law.

There will always be pros and cons or consistent or inconsistent factors that can be surmised when analyzing one's religious exemption and that it why the whole concept of being questioned about it is rotten, reeks of impropriety and must be declared as legally improper and unjust. If you state your religious exemption is a fraud or fabrication then it is obviously invalid however, absent your admission of putting forward an untrue religious belief it is legally impossible to determine that your religious exemption is invalid or not sincere. You can find religion at a moment notice and your past actions should not be allowed or used to refute your present religion or religious conviction. Your religion is between you and GOD; not the overzealous, obtrusive State! Only you can deem your religious belief wrong or right thus, others denying your religious belief is a fraud. The State or the school sanctioned by the State to decide upon your religious exemption is favoring one religion over another or is favoring one belief over another and is without relevant or material evidence is crucifying people's religious beliefs. There is no evidence that can prove belief; there is only the belief itself and/or faith. Refusal to be vaccinated is only evidence that you refuse to be vaccinated; belief can neither be proved or disproved. When GOD enters you is not important; it is that GOD is in you that is all-important!

The States are not all on the same page when it comes to exemptions however, all States must allow for Religious Exemption because it is considered part of Freedom of Religion which is protected under the Constitution even though a few states do not. All 50 states have legislation requiring childhood vaccination for students. All school immunization laws grant exemptions to children for medical reasons if they can prove it with doctors notes etc. Currently, 18 states allow philosophical exemptions for those who object to immunizations because of personal, moral or other beliefs. Yes, there are people claiming religious exemption as a last resort to prevent their children from potential harm from vaccination. Sometime the law is an ass and placing people in an untenable position with a callous vaccination mandate is making people seek religious exemptions however, although there may be some that call upon religion because they feel they have no choice; the questioning of these people about it must be declared illegal, unamerican and unconstitutional. It is impossible to determine sincerity without an admission of it and the very act of questioning it violates the requirement of Separation of Church and State.

Those that benefit financially from mandated vaccination, with thousands of lobbyists do not want you to be free to follow your religion if it means it decreases profit from vaccination. Be acutely aware, freedom of religion has already been destroyed as had occurred by the SB 277 mal-enactment in California. Mississippi and West Virginia are also, not abiding by the Constitution in that they do not recognize religious exemption. Italy and France now no longer have religious exemption for vaccinations. We must realize that our essential freedoms are under attack and that this loss of liberty has caused vaccines to be chemically unsafe. Please, help the charity, SAFER vaccines do something about it! If, The People, cannot refuse and unwanted vaccine chemical concoction and/or if we are not free to litigate against these vaccine makers then they can put any nasty, unhealthy or unnatural to the biology chemicals that it wants in our children's vital vaccine supply! On a positive note, as of July 2017 there are two bills that if passed will likely help end the above unconstitutionality, one bill in the Assembly, A8123a and one bill in the Senate, S8141c. Freedom of religious vaccination exemptions prompts vaccines to be produced with less or no unnatural to the body chemicals and thus, not as religiously objectionable! If you are prepared and present your religious belief in an organized way it could be granted. You also, need to be FREE to REFUSE if you deem a vaccine dangerous!

Imagine being in front of a fault-finding committee that has authority to either grant your religious exemption or deny it. You may surmise that they are out to get you and that they have agenda to discredit and invalidate your religion or religious belief that prevents you from vaccinating your children. The intrusion upon what you consider most private is beyond painful and disheartening, but you feel you must submit to save your children from being taken from you and injected against your will and religion. You own that it is GOD's will that prevents the vaccine chemicalization injections and that your will is GOD's will. If your religion is ignored or your religious conviction is rendered void or not worthy of religious exemption you fear that you will be left no choice but to sin so, to avoid being a mandated vaccination law breaker or societal outcast. Your intelligence tells you that not only would it be a sin to vaccinate but also, the unnatural to human biology chemicals in vaccines will be destructive to your children's vital biochemistry needed for optimal health. Perhaps you know a family that refused vaccination after their religious exemption was denied and consequently, child services were called in and took the child from the parents to inject the child and thereby, traumatized and made the child hysterical. Even though it was against the family's religion and against the parents will or understanding that the vaccine was too dangerous to inject, child services forced the injection upon their hysterical little girl. With the one-sided determination of religious exemption and the susceptibility to being enforced to be vaccinated under a for profit vaccination mandate law we are too susceptible and need to implement the TWO STEPS OF CORRECTION that SAFER Vaccines charity totally supports.

People are being forced to choose between Divine law and that of man-made mandated vaccination law when their religion or religious exemption is denied! Knowing that your child might be ripped out of your arms and whisked away to suffer an unwanted vaccine chemicalization injection if your religious exemption id denied if you still refuse vaccination is not merely, putting people between a rock and a hard place; it often makes people violate their religion. People do not want to be treated as if they are law breakers or dubbed a neglector of their children for not vaccinating and so, they cave in even though it is against one's religion to vaccinate and may bring the wrath of GOD down upon them for doing so. The coercion or abuse goes further when parents realize their children are being exposed to the known and unknown negative to health consequences of being subjected to unnatural to human biology chemicaliztion from an injected vaccine. Parents are also, strongly coerced into vaccinating their children and violating their religion since they feel they have no choice in the matter because their perfectly healthy unvaccinated children are not allowed to enter school to receive their fundamental education. Perfectly healthy children, in no need of medical intervention are being enforced to be injected against the will and religion of both parents and children. Vaccination mandate and denial of religious exemption violates the person who is vaccinated, violates the parental Right to protect children from what they determine is a chemicalization harm and violates religion of those claiming religious exemption. THERE MUST BE LIBERTY

TO REJECT INJECTIONS! No liberty to reject injections and Religious Exemption being readily denied and not holding vaccine producers to the flames of negligence law when its vaccines induce injury instills less vaccine quality control and tends to make vaccines unsafe with chemicals for profit. DO NOT RELIQUISH YOUR RELIGIOUS CONVICTION AGAINST BEING VACCINATED!

Having one's religion or religious belief questioned or analyzed for determination of religious exemption from vaccination mandated law is fraught with illegality. It is not a cleansing inspection; it is an attempt to discredit you and disavow your belief. Through arbitrary and capricious methodology, they miraculously, determine if one's religious belief is sincere or if the religious exemption is valid; this religion witch hunt must be declared against the law. Surely, if a person seeking a religious exemption goes before these government sanctioned fault finders or truth squad then the person is really facing a firing squad that dismisses one's religion or religious belief as unworthy or not sincere and thereby, voids the exemption or never allows for it. They may ask is your religious conviction is a long held one not to be vaccinated as if it could factor in determining the granting of a religious exemption. Checking sincerity based upon how long one has had one's belief is inappropriate. A long-term held religious belief and a short-term belief must be given equal weight; people must be taken for their word after all, it is their belief. Separation of Church and State forbids this line of questioning at any level! No free practicing religious American should be required to confess their private religious beliefs and moreover, no one should be questioned if their belief is sincere. What is controlling whether it is legal or not legal is the fact that one's body is one's temple (1 Corinthians 6:19-20, NIV) *Therefore honor God with your bodies* thus, government's mandate to vaccinate is a violation of Separation of Church and State and thereby, unconstitutional. Secure Freedom of Religion!

The mandated vaccination law and the interrogation into religious exemption are unworkable and illegal because the Constitutional requirement that our Government must not favor one religion over another and/or establish one religion over another is violated by favoring those with religious exemption not to be vaccinated with school entrance and at the same time denying entrance to those who's religion does not require a religious exemption if they remain unvaccinated. Those that do not have the required religious exemption and remain unvaccinated are prejudiced for not having the right religion by not allowing school entrance or rather, government by its act of allowing school entrance of unvaccinated children with the right religious belief is the act of establishing one religion over another or favoring one religion over another based upon belief. The act of different treatment based upon religious belief is the establishment of one religion over another. The act of basing school admittance based upon religion establishes one religion over another. The act of treating unvaccinated children differently based upon one's religious belief or religion is the government establishing a religion over another religion. The act of allowing school entrance for unvaccinated based upon religious exemption is establishing that religion as superior, favored or as required. By one's religious belief one person may enter school and one may not enter school crosses the line from justice to injustice. The imperfection or injustice of manmade law should never infringe upon your religion.

In addition, the Mandated vaccination law and religious exemption viability are erroneous and unconstitutional because those who do not have the special favored religion must suffer an unwanted vaccination whereas, those with the government approved religious exemption do not. The law favors or rewards those who have the requisite religion with not enforcing vaccination whereas, those without the government approved religion must suffer an unwanted vaccination, it prejudices the non-favored religions that are not vaccinated with enforced vaccinations otherwise no school entrance. This special treatment favors one religion over another and/or coerces one to be vaccinated. This is a violation of the requirement of Separation of Church and State and is against the Establishment Clause.

The Fifth Amendment and the Fourteenth Amendment each contain a due process clause. The due process clause acts as a safeguard from arbitrary denial of life, liberty, or property by the government outside the sanction of law. The arbitrary and capricious questioning by school boards about one's religious exemption violates procedural due process and just how the school is to determine if a person's religious faith or conviction is sincere or valid violates substantive due process in that the law is vague. In addition, Equal Protection is violated because the people are being treated differently under the law. People are being treated differently in that certain people must be vaccinated while others do not have to be vaccinated. It is analogous to allowing some people to have an exemption to go through a red light while other citizens may not. The concept that by religion you can go through a red light or not be subject to the mandated vaccination law violates fairness, equality and equality; it indicates vaccination mandates are unworkable. Perhaps you do not want to be vaccinated or do not want your children to be vaccinated because you do not agree with the concept of injecting o putting in a disease to prevent a disease or perhaps you have determined that it is against GOD's will; either way, a FREE AMERICAN should not be enforced to vaccinate against their will and/or religious belief.

There is no "rational basis" to a "legitimate State purpose" to require or sanction the interrogation or questioning of an individual's religion or religious belief. The insidious requirement of Religious Exemption and its calculated denial has become the cornerstone that Freedom of Religion must hinge upon; it either allows the Free Exercise of Religion or forbids it. Exemption or lack of exemption warps the ideology of "justice" resulting in "just for us", if you have the special religion or approved religious belief to ward off vaccination. Only those found to have the special religion or religious belief get the golden stamp of approval of a bonified approved religion and/or exemption from vaccination. Denial of religious exemptions are based upon arbitrary and capricious methodology and the approval of certain special religious convictions fails the requirement of fundamental principles of liberty and justice. The questioning and the authority to decide if one's religious belief is sincere or worthy of exemption crosses a forbidden line; it is illegal under the Constitution. In addition, there is no balancing test in place, anything is asked. GOVERNMENT SANCTIONED RELIGIOUS

EXEMPTION IS GOVERNMENT SANCTIONED RELIGION; mandated vaccination is impermissible with or without Religious Exemption. SAFER Vaccines, the charity is acting to correct any law that minimizes or deters the accomplishment of SAFER vaccines and thereby, protect the basic Rights and welfare of people.

Only you have dominion over your religious belief; no one else should dictate or control it; even if they doubt your belief. Only your doubt can prevent you from moving mountains! However, no one should have to move mountains to obtain a religious exemption! Merely, because they doubt you do not let it cause you to be deterred or severe you from your religious belief; do not let others severe you or detach you from what it is, you believe. Stand strong in your religious belief; defy what is against your religion, do not be made to kneel to what you know is a vaccine evil or violation of your religion. If vaccination is not truly against your religion then by all means, contemplate vaccination but, always protect your children from too dangerous to inject vaccine chemicalization injections! At least, be religious about protecting your children from all dangers! If GOD tells you to not allow an injection, then that must be enough for a Religious Exemption. If you think GOD would conclude that the vaccine is harmful then this should be considered a valid reason to obtain a Religious Exemption. If you think that a vaccine is too harmful or has unnatural to human biology chemicals and you are religious about protecting your children then this also, must be considered valid reason to obtain a Religious Exemption. Rights such as, procreation or liberty to protect your children from what a parent considers a harm are Rights which come from GOD, they are unalienable Rights; not to be given up or suppressed.

Remember, obtaining a Religious Exemption is not about mere belief or philosophy; it is about your Religious belief in what GOD commands and teaches. The Bible instructs, "Beware lest anyone cheat you through philosophy and empty deceit..."(Colossians 2:8-10), this applies in the instant case of the mere philosophy of vaccination or its supposed benefits and the deceit surrounding of why it is mandated and being enforced upon people and why you are being overburdened by questions regarding your religion or Religious belief in relying on the power of GOD and forbids vaccination. You are not a mere robot that automatically vaccinates; you are one with GOD and seek personal stability in the Holy Spirit, Romans 15:13 teaches, "Now may the GOD of hope fill you with all joy and peace in believing, that you abound in hope by the power of the Holy Spirit". Your religion may not permit you to allow your children to suffer a vaccination!

The deceit or evil that has befallen so many and/or made vaccines turn into a method and madness of injecting tiny babies, little infants and small children with vaccines that are laced with unnatural to human biology chemicals is spawned by the self-serving total liability shield obtained for Big Pharma that protect it or rather its unconscionable profiteering even when its vaccines are accused of inducing injury to those vaccinated. In addition, the deceit and evil of mandating vaccination for profit that egregiously violate parents GOD given Right to protect their children in that the erroneous mandate bypasses or make informed consent or rather informed DENIAL of vaccination a moot point or a none requirement to give a vaccination. The above-mentioned deceit and/or evil has rendered vaccines chemically unsafe in that chemicals for profit not safety is in vaccines; making vaccines too dangerous to inject. The departure of law enumeration from GOD or not centering law enactment around GOD's will has rendered law impure. In today's age where our law-making edifices have taken a sharp turn away from GOD whereas, our founding fathers prayed before they went about their lawmaking business. Indeed, law was once predicated on goodness, on purity, on GOD; it is no longer! GODIFY your decision about vaccination and do not fall victim to the cunning craftiness of people in their deceitful schemes. GODIFY your life and you will be healthy and happy!

Deceit or evil permeates throughout the involuntary vaccination system; it has both the vaccine manufacturer and doctors that inject its vaccines above the law in that they cannot be held accountable and liable for vaccine induced injuries. Because of this unprecedented wrongful corporate protection children are much more likely to be chemically compromised by vaccine injections; our children are not being protected from negligent production of vaccines. Children are more vulnerable to injury because there is a lot less incentive to assure vaccine safety. Since, there is no accountability and liability due to the total liability shield, producers of vaccines concentration is not on safety therefore, they tend to put whatever chemicals in its vaccines that make vaccines most profitable. It is of utmost importance that parents are given all the chemicals that are in vaccines before contemplation of injection for parents are rendered breathless and devastated after the fact. To be manipulated into vaccination by not being given essential information of chemical content or being given disinformation that vaccines are "absolutely safe" is dishonesty to the extreme, an evil; to be mandated to vaccinate especially, if the vaccine has any unnatural to human biology chemicals is an act of aggression against your children and visits them with evil. Full disclosure and liberty to decide what will flow throughout your body and blood combats deceit and evil; if you know in your heart that GOD would want it this way then you do deserve a Religious Exemption. By the grace of GOD given parental Right you are FREE to reject injections especially, if you know the vaccine is laced with unnatural to human biology chemicals!

We have all kinds of freedoms however, the liberty to decide what is best for one's children and to be completely FREE to live by the Word of GOD are without question among the greatest of liberties. To be in self-control of what can or cannot enter our bodies is off the chart when it comes to Rights. It is of supreme importance to life and liberty, it is indispensable to control what will or will not be injected into our very own vital blood chemistries or systems. Parents by GOD given Right must have this most basic of fundamental freedom to decide if vaccines will benefit their children and/or be accepted or are too dangerous to inject. Many good souls are blessed with GOD directing them.

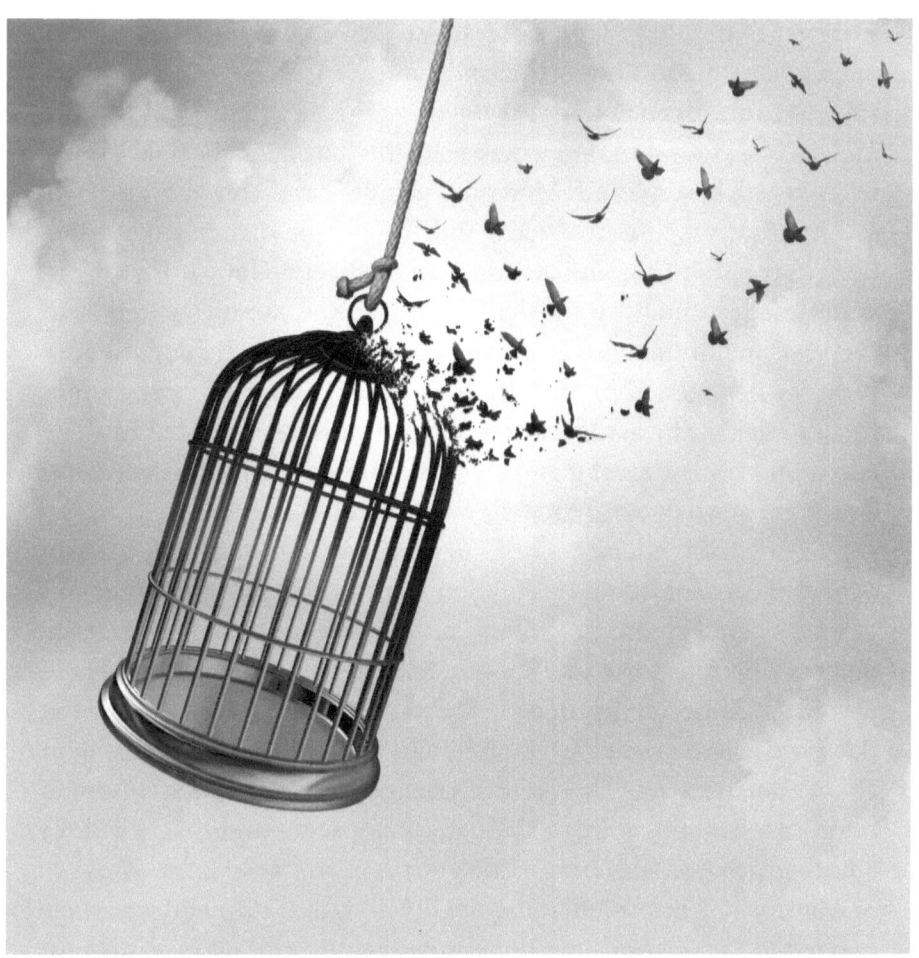

BE FREE TO REJECT INJECTIONS!

This vaccine chemical content free-for-all has taken place because vaccine manufacturers are not subject to the safety precautions that are instilled by negligence lawsuit susceptibility under negligence law or from informed consent/DENIAL and/or liberty to refuse vaccine chemicalization and thereby, places our children in grave danger, at risk of suffering an imperfect, unsafe vaccine and/or a vaccine that carries unnatural to human biology chemicals. Children are in jeopardy of vaccines made more for profit and not with safety as, its number one priority; safety is not a must, profits are! There is a danger of division in allowing the vaccine industry to depart from negligence law; to have it that our children's vaccine supply is not subject to negligence law and unconscionably to not hold vaccine makers to a good standard which is instilled by negligence law is not in children's best interest. Moreover, people reasonably automatically assume that vaccine producers and the doctor that inoculates are held to the tradition and standard of negligence law. If the public is not made acutely aware that those involved are an exception to the legal requirement of being held accountable or liable for injury from its negligence or that those injured from a vaccine cannot litigate against the actual causer of injury, it is deceitful because the common people expect it and are not made aware. This is deceit and deceit are another word for evil; be not made subjected to it!

The deceit renders you without pertinent knowledge to make an educated decision about vaccination, it leaves one purposely ignorant of what chemicals are in vaccines or that vaccine producers and the doctors who inject the vaccines are not held accountable and liable if your children are injured by the vaccination. Deceit makes the decision to vaccinate discernable and thereby, makes judgement about vaccine safety or whether vaccination is in one's children's best interest impossible, inadequate or improper and that is evil. In addition, what is alarming is that without the auspices and safety precautions of informed consent/DENIAL and no negligence law applied to vaccinations, producers of vaccines will not be exuberant about assuring our children are not unnecessarily exposed to unnatural to the human biology chemicals. Such, chemicals have been found in vaccines and remain in vaccines. If your religion teaches to treat your body as a temple or that you must subject oneself to unnatural to human biology vaccine injections, then do claim a Religious Exemption! Does your religion protect you and your children from such evil? Perhaps, you will join the enlightened and let GOD protect you from such, folly! Become religious about health; do not violate your body with an evil! If you determine injecting a vaccine chemicalization is an evil, then you must be FREE to do whatever is necessary to prevent your children from being visited or violated with what you deem is a CHEMICALIZATION EVIL.

The leadership vacuum has allowed the self-serving protection of Big Pharma and left our children vulnerable to strictly profiteering decisions. The purity of our children's delicate chemistries has been blundered as a result. It is deceitful that they keep the public unaware that they cannot litigate against a vaccine producer for a negligently produced vaccine or the doctor who injected the injurious vaccine when children are injured by the vaccine chemicalization. The fact, that that neither pay a single cent to compensate for an injury caused by an injurious vaccination has been kept from the super majority of parents and to keep parents in the dark about it is dishonesty on steroids. If parents were made acutely aware of the truth, they would not be made to blindly trust that vaccines are safe and would be much more precautious about vaccination. You should know that having unnatural to human biology chemicals n vaccines is so bad for you that you should be required to sign a document that you have been made well aware of the fact, and require that you sign that no liability can be sought against the manufacturer of the vaccine or against the doctor that injects it; then and only then will the evil lies and/or deceit will cease. But, always remember that if you are religious about treating your body as, a temple by not exposing yourself or family to unnatural to the body chemicalization then your religion can and will set you FREE!

Not being subject to being accountable or liable for vaccine induced injuries there is much greater tendency to put chemicals for profit in vaccines that are unnatural to human biology chemicals and this chemicalization causes abnormal reactions. Most parents would agree that it is a lie and deceitful to state vaccines are safe and an egregious lie to state that vaccines are "absolutely safe" under the above set of circumstances. Also, most parents are unaware or do not realize until it is brought to their attention that informed consent/DENIAL is not required under the mandated vaccination law and that without the ability to legally refuse a mandated vaccination it allows producers of vaccines to put whatever chemicals it wants or that makes vaccines most profitable despite the fact, they it is unhealthy or has no benefit to those vaccinated. In combination it makes for evil to be visited upon your children but, you may have the saving grace of having a religion that forbids this evil from visiting your children! Everyone knows that money is a root of evil; if mandated vaccinations were not profitable it would not be mandated! A reason why thiomersal, the MERCURY derivative preservative was put in childhood vaccines was that it produced more profit to do so; that is evil!

As far as, any unaccountable vaccine producer or doctor that treats our children wrong by producing a vaccine that is laced with unnatural to human biology chemicals or inoculates a vaccine with such, chemicals when it is possible to achieve SAFER vaccines or have less if not any unnatural chemicals in vaccines they should be fired and made to pay severally for compromising children's vital to health and life perfected chemistries. The saving grace of GOD can protect you from such, abnormalizing to one's biochemistry vaccine concoctions if your religious conviction does not permit it however, it is a shame that we must have fall onto our knees in religion to avoid having our children's from being chemically compromised. The TWO STEPS OF CORRECTION that the charity SAFER Vaccines backs is to achieve SAFER vaccines and thereby, secure SAFER CHILDREN; is the right way, the best way. Hold vaccine producers liable for vaccine induced injuries and make vaccination based upon informed consent/DENIAL. Thank GOD for your belief in GOD for if all else fails, the power of GOD and His inspired Constitution will protect you. The power of GOD is more than enough to protect your family from childhood disease for GOD can even raise the dead; His power is omnipotent. Luke 7:14-15, God said, "Young man, I say to you, get up!" The dead man sat up and Jesus gave him back to his mother. Having the limitless power of GOD on your side do you need vaccination? Do you think injecting vaccine chemicalization is the desecration of your body and blood in violation of GOD?

Lie and deceit that vaccines were "absolutely safe" is wonton dishonesty and wrongful conduct that allowed the Bill which unconscionably renders both the vaccine producers and doctors whom administer vaccines a total liability shield impervious to litigation surrounding vaccine induced injuries. Congressmen and Senators were duped into passing the self-serving and grossly inappropriate total liability shield because they were repetitively, told the blatant lie that vaccines were "absolutely safe". It is deceit that vaccines are safe if they contain unnatural to human biology chemicals and the Vaccination Court using taxpayer dollars awarding over a Billion dollars to those injured by vaccines proves just how unsafe vaccines really are. The involuntary vaccination delivery system is egregiously unjust and is based upon evil. We must be FREE not to visit our children with evil especially, if GOD has warned us not to rely on it. Our nation is based upon religious liberty; we desperately need our religion to protect us!

Those whom seek Religious Exemption from vaccination can have confidence in their religious belief that all you need for health is GOD or that to rely on injections of vaccine chemicalization is a sin. Do not be made to conform your religion to vaccination mandate or kneel to conformity. Align yourself with GOD; not social influence or attitudes of mass behavior. ISAIAH 41:10, "So do not fear, for I am with you; do not be dismayed; for I am your GOD. I will strengthen you and help you; I will uphold you with my righteous right hand." So, when acting to stay healthy or when fighting off disease or preventing vaccination that is against your religion put your faith in GOD, be strong and know the Almighty is with you and so, put the full armor of GOD on. EPHESIANS 6:11, "Put the full armor of GOD, so that you can take a stand against the devil's schemes." EPHESIANS 6:13-18, "Therefore put on the full armor of GOD, so that when the day of evil comes," (the threat of childhood disease and/or the threat of unnatural to the body vaccine chemicalization) "you may be able to stand your ground, and after you have done everything, to stand. Stand firm then, with the belt of truth buckled around your waste, with the breastplate of righteousness in place, and with your feet fitted with the readiness that comes from gospel of peace, in addition to all this, take up the shield of faith, with which you can extinguish all the flaming arrows of the evil one." (disease, Autism and/or vaccination) "Take the helmet of salvation and the sword of the Spirit, which is the word of GOD. And pray in the Spirit on all occasions with all kinds of prayers and requests." Salvation is the deliverance from sin and its consequences brought about by faith so, keep to your faith by obtaining a Religious Exemption. ROMANS

11:36, "For from him and through him and for him are all things. To him be the glory forever! Amen." Good overcomes evil but you must first recognize what it is that is evil.

GOD protects us from evil; GOD delivers us from evil. Do you recognize that injecting vaccines which contain unnatural to human biology chemicals as an evil or that relying upon or injecting man-made vaccine concoctions when your children are perfectly healthy as, evil that is against GOD's Law? If you have asked yourself, would Jesus or GOD submit to injections of vaccine chemicalization and the answer is "NO" then if you believe in Jesus or GOD you must not submit to vaccination. What if you just now ask the question and just now recognize that you have a religious conviction against vaccination; surely, you should be entitled to obtain a Religious Exemption from having to submit under the mandated vaccination law!

MANY HAVE OBTAINED DEVINE KNOWLEDGE OR JUST PLAIN OLD, NORMAL TRUTH; THAT TO INJECT CHEMICALS THAT HAVE BEEN FOUND IN VACCINES CAUSE ABNORMAL BIOCHEMICAL REACTIONS AND IS AGAINST GOD'S TRUTH. WHETHER OR NOT INJECTING UNNATURAL TO HUMAN BIOLOGY AND FOREIGN TO NORMAL BIOCHEMISTRY IS A VIOLATION AGIANST GOD IS ENTIRELY UP TO HOW YOU INTERPRET WHAT JESUS OR GOD WOULD DECREE WHICH MEANS; IF YOU DEEM IT AGAINST YOUR RELIGION YOU MUST BE AFFORDED A RELIGIOUS EXEMPTION! WHETHER YOUR RELIGIOUS BELIEF OR RELIGION IS OR IS NOT A COMMON RELIGIOUS CONVICTION MUST HAVE NO BARRING ON A RELIGIOUS EXEMPTION DETERMINATION. YOUR RELIGIOUS UNDERSTANDING OR SPIRITUAL BELIEF OR WHAT MAKES RELIGIOUS COMMON SENCE TO YOU; IS WHAT SHOULD MATTER FOR RELIGIOUS EXEMPTION!

If there is a herd mentality to be vaccinated or that it is convenient to submit to vaccinations should not influence your religious decision on vaccination nor, should it be a factor in Religious Exemption obtainment or denial. If vaccines are not needed or should not be depended upon according to your GOD or your religion; then

Religious Exemption should be granted. If you determine that a vaccine chemicalization is not safe because it is against GOD's Law or what YOU THINK GOD WOULD DO OR WHAT GOD WANTS YOU TO DO; then you must be afforded a Religious Exemption. If your religion dictates that your sacred blood chemistry would be defiled and thereby, your religion violated you must be granted a Religious Exemption. If you think GOD deems that a vaccine chemicalization denatures or causes abnormal bioreactions or has is not required by GOD to be healthy then you might consider it your religious belief that your religion or understanding of GOD's Laws forbids you choose to penetrate your body and/or biology with vaccination. BE FREE TO CONTROL THE CHEMISTRY OF YOUR BODY AND BLOOD THE WAY YOU THINK GOD WANTS! If vaccination does not coincide with your religion, reject it!

What cannot be proved is that GOD cannot do what you say GOD can do. If your religious belief is that if you follow GOD's Law and/or strictly rely upon GOD for health you and your children will be healthy and conversely, if you violate your religion by not strictly relying upon GOD by injecting vaccine chemicalizations; you and your children may not remain healthy and GOD may not protect you and thereby, being diagnosed with Autism becomes possible. The power of prayer taps into the power of GOD and has caused miraculous healings. Those who were deathly ill have miraculously, become healthy through prayer and asking GOD for his divine intervention. We must be FREE to rely upon GOD's intervention and not forced to rely upon man-made medical intervention or be caused to sin in the eyes of GOD by being caused not to strictly rely upon GOD. A too high number of people are taking drugs and too many unnecessarily take an army of drugs or vaccines when many people think all they really need is GOD. It is no coincidence that drug dependency and an increased need for operations coincide. There are those that think because we have moved away from GOD and depend more upon the medical intervention of vaccination that an Autism epidemic is plaquing our children. The key to prevent Autism is to achieve SAFER vaccines and/or allowing people the FREE EXERCISE of their religion. Intelligent designed inventions that aid mankind must not be pushed upon us or jammed down our throats; and must not force one to violate their religion!

An aspect of religion is to safeguard you against evil and if according to your religion it is evil to inject vaccine chemicalizations; you must not be commanded by a callous, nonpermissive law to violate your religion or Free Exercise of it! Merely, because orthodox medicine says vaccination is a must or that the world conforms to undergo vaccination; you must not be coerced or enforced to conform if GOD or your religion tells you not to. ROMANS 12:1-2, "Therefore, I urge you, brothers and sisters, in view of GOD's mercy, to offer your bodies as a living sacrifice, holy and pleasing to GOD – this is your true and proper worship. Do not conform to the pattern of this world but be transformed by the renewing of your mind. Then you will be able to test and approve what GOD's will is --- his good, pleasing and perfect will." Therefore, let your religion conform you; do not conform to laws that violate your religion or dictate vaccination if it is against what you deem GOD wants! Stand strong against what violates your religion; do not succumb to sin! Acknowledge GOD and pray for wisdom to best protect your children.

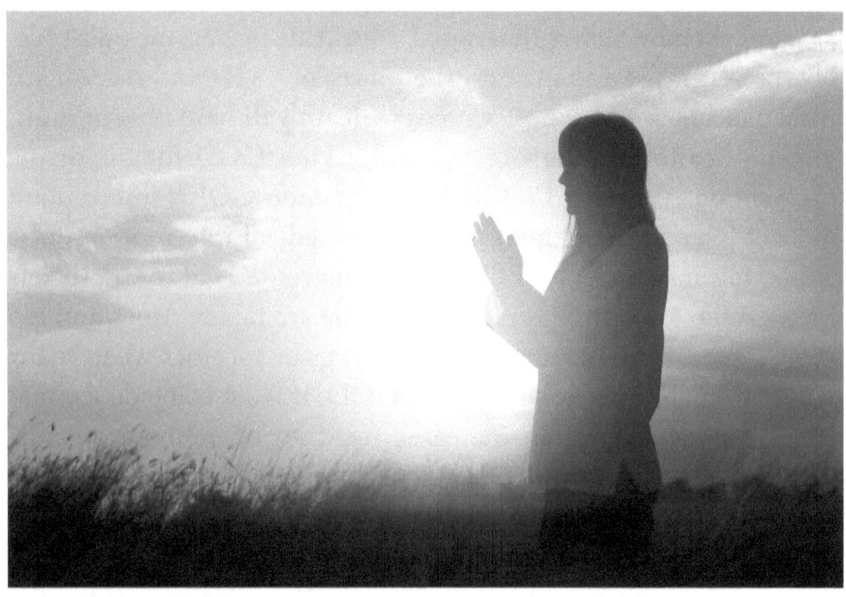

BE FREE TO STRICTLY RELY UPON GOD!

Pray for health and it will be yours; pray; if you pray that your children are healthy, they will be. ROMANS 12:17, Prayer is the channel GOD uses so that His strength can flow into our lives." So, continually pray and you will be protected by GOD; pray no harm will come to you and your family; believe that you have received GOD's protection from serious illness and it will be given you and thereby, no need to brake from your religion and suffer an unwanted vaccine injection! Prayer is not foreign to our nation in fact, our nation was based upon it. The very first Congress was initiated with a prayer and as part of the prayer the following words had set Congress on the path to do good in the eyes of the Lord.

"Be thou present, O God of wisdom, and DIRECT THE COUNCILS of this honorable assembly; enable them to settle things on the best and surest foundation. That the scene of blood may be speedily closed; that order, harmony and peace maybe effectually restored, and truth and justice, religion and piety, prevail and flourish among the people. PRESERVE THE HEALTH of their bodies and vigor of their minds...." and so, once upon a religious time before Congress went about making law all lawmakers were centered in GOD. You can bet your last dollar that every single member of Congress would have easily obtained a Religious Exemption from vaccination had the need arose. Our nation began on prayer when the Continental Congress came to Philadelphia for the first time in September 1774.

There was no opposition over starting Congress each time by praying to GOD however, there was opposition for having to pray together with all the different religions having to pray together. The impasse was broken when the revolutionary, Sam Adams, declared, "I am no bigot. I can pray with any man who loves his God and loves his country." Today our Congressmen do not start their duty to preserve the Constitution and make laws that are supposed to serve the public, with prayer; and we are all suffering for it. So, prayer is not foreign to how government operates or how it masters our lives; what is foreign, is that today our religion is being placed on trial or rather under question when we are coerced into having to do so to obtain a religious Exemption. Mandated vaccination law is an abomination as, is the wrongful inquiry into Religious belief. Denial of people's Religious Exemption from unwanted vaccine chemicalization injection is unconstitutional. Secure Freedom of Religion!

When it comes to combating disease or remaining healthy your religion may have it that GOD gave you an immune system that is powerful enough however, if for any reason it is determined that it is not powerful enough, you know GOD is on your side; all you must do is pray to GOD. GOD is ALL POWERFUL so, if you pray for strength or resistance against disease and have faith in GOD THE ALL POWERFULL, that you have been given what you ask for and have no doubt in your heart of GOD's blessing then be assured that what you pray for is yours. We do not have enough built in immune response or mental energy to withstand all the diseases out there or to withstand all the temptations facing us, and no one can live 100% righteously in our evil age apart from the power of Christ, the Holy Spirit and/or GOD so, it is your religious belief to put GOD on the thrown and to rely on His omnipotent power to be healthy that overpowers all disease. Certainly, man-made medical intervention is fallible, does not achieve what it is meant to and too often causes illness or iatrogenic disease. If you believe in fighting childhood disease by being strong in the power of GOD, overcoming weakness with unstoppable strength; believing that GOD's power is an overcoming power then you certainly, deserve a Religious Exemption. You are FREE to rely upon GOD for health and throw yourself at the feet of GOD for health and to be strong in the power of His might. Remain faithful to GOD to be healthy, Acts 1:8 says, "But you shall receive power when the Holy Spirit has come upon you; and you shall be a witness to Me." Do not be a witness to vaccination if your religion does not allow for it; and do not let them deny what you hold true in religion!

Our Creator is in the most important documents that America was founded upon however, we live in times were we no longer use the documents, nor do we base our law strictly upon them; we need to have GOD's Law as the basis of all law. We have moved away from Nature's Laws or GOD's Laws; we need to GODIFY in order, to secure our great nation. The Declaration of Independence has GOD as, its corner stone, having words, "the Laws of Nature and of Nature's God entitle....", however, this most important founding document is hardly mentioned today or when it is mentioned they unwisely, leave out referring to GOD. Years gone by, school used to require testing based upon one's knowledge or understanding of the Declaration and the Constitution; today most students are ignorant about the words and principles of these documents that this nation must be based upon. These principles percolated and became well known during colony times. It was nothing new to the minds of the colonists when these documents came to be.

History shows that before these documents came into existence, the fundamentals of the words and principles memorialized in the founding documents were taught, often preached, almost daily by the preachers during colonial time; the words and principles are older than America itself and is the basis of why the founding fathers rebelled to forge America. So, in contemplation of injecting vaccine chemicalization; do be sure it coincides with the words and principles set forth in the Declaration and Constitution. Vaccination is a major life decision that can majorly effect health! Those with the needed belief in their GOD know; GOD is bigger than vaccination; GOD is enough to conquer what vaccines are designed for; so, be not deterred, do execute your Freedom of Religion. Be proactive in your faith and do seek to obtain your rightful Religious Exemption! Expect a flood of GOD's favor, GOD is sufficient; rely on Him and rest in GOD's promise! If your religion has you living in victory, as a victor, not a victim because GOD's grace is upon you; with faith there is no need for vaccination. Do not let others disbelief rob you of your belief; do not be prevented from having GOD be your protector; obtain the needed Religious Exemption!

These most important documents that America was founded upon made it essential that our law protect our GOD given and/or Natural Rights; recognizing there is a GOD and that Rights come from GOD; grants us moral laws and requires that the law be made only with the consent of the people. When you leave GOD outside of your law making or render public education devoid of GOD; the principles of this great nation are lost and what holds this nation together begins to crumble and our Rights become afflicted and violated. In the beginning and until recent times almost 100% of the people voted for the President but now a pitiful percentage of people vote. People because they were taught about the founding documents and GOD's law felt it their obligation to vote. Today we are in the mess we are in because we have removed GOD from law making or made GOD unessential to how we act and live. It is faltered to the point that our Religion or religious beliefs are being questioned, challenged and too often dismissed as invalid. What is extremely disturbing as, of recent times or generation is, that we have taken GOD out of the equation in our law making, in children's schooling and in our everyday lives! Some think we are doomed for doing so; I say, it is high time to bring GOD into our lives; let us start by ending tyranny against Freedom of Religion by stopping religious belief scrutiny, questioning or challenging to obtain a Religious Exemption from vaccination.

The Declaration of Independence has it that GOD is at the center of our lives and if our government which, is meant to serve the People does instead, do the People a disservice by violating unalienable Rights "endowed by the Creator", then Government needs to be corrected to secure our inalienable Rights. There is the "Right of the People to alter or to abolish it, and to institute new Government", according to the Declaration. It is written, "We hold these truths to be self-evident, that all men are created equal, that they are endowed by their Creator with certain unalienable Rights, that among these are Life, Liberty and the pursuit of Happiness.--That to secure these rights, Governments are instituted among Men, deriving their just powers from the consent of the governed, --That whenever any Form of Government becomes destructive of these ends, it is the Right of the People to alter or to abolish it, and to institute new Government, laying its foundation on such principles and organizing its powers in such form, as to them shall seem most likely to affect their Safety and Happiness." Your Right to follow your religious belief to strictly rely upon GOD and thereby, not to be injected with vaccines is an "unalienable Right" that is "self-evident". True religious liberty does not require a Religious Exemption! To forbid one to live by their religion by enforcing vaccine chemicalization against their religious belief or to question or challenge one's religious belief and/or require a Religious Exemption or refuse to give one is the establishment of an absolute Tyranny over religion!

I consider the following spiritual words unlock the secret of life and success; the most important on point verses from the Bible which, make it crystal clear that what you pray for and have faith in will occur. If you pray to GOD for your children to stay healthy or become healthy they most certainly, will if your belief is resolute. In the book of Mark, chapter 11 verse 22, Jesus answered, "Have faith in GOD" and Mark chapter 11 verse 23, "Truly I tell you, if anyone says to this mountain 'Go throw yourself into this sea,' and does not doubt in their heart but believes that what they say will happen, it will be done for them. Therefore, I tell you whatever you ask for in prayer, believe that you have received it, and it will be yours." Please, note that you must believe that you have already "received" what it is that you pray for. Do not be deprived of living a life under the rule of GOD and do protect your children according to your religious belief!

You may have religious belief that if you pray for a blessing and in all your heart do not doubt that it will occur and believe what you ask GOD for you have received then you may apply this GOD's truth to health; so, consider making this Law of GOD part of your religion. If it is part of your religion, then Freedom of Religion allows one not to rely upon vaccinations; even if it is mandated by mere man-made law. Vaccinations have commonly scared people, caused signs and symptoms of injury, distorted the natural biochemistry and spawned abnormal to the body reactions, with its unnatural to human biology chemicals; it is no wonder that to inject such, denaturing is against GOD or people's religious beliefs! People must not be forced to commit a sin if vaccination is against GOD's law rather, "Have faith in GOD"; and procure a righteous Religious Exemption! Be FREE to GODIFY your decision about vaccination through Freedom of Religion and obtain a Religious Exemption. There must be liberty to rely upon only GOD to sustain perfect health or for health and not be enforced to vaccinate! Religious Exemption from vaccination assure Liberty to rely upon GOD and not mandated vaccination; GODIFY!

If you do not take a stand against what you deem is a too dangerous to inject vaccine based upon the logic that to inject your child would be an act of child abuse by chemicalization then by all means, do perfect your Religious Exemption. A baby having to adapt, respond or react to the antigens in a vaccine is a difficult task in itself; to also, suffer the baby with unnatural to human biology chemicalization is much too abusive; as it subjects the baby to abnormal internal reactions and/or abnormality. The charity SAFER Vaccines' mission is to secure SAFER vaccines for all our children's benefit and welfare however, the charity is strongly supportive of Religious Freedom and/or Religious Exemption. SAFER Vaccines charity is pro- voluntary vaccination that is based upon TWO STEPS OF CORRECTION to GET THE CHEMICALS OUT.

If vaccines were not an affliction upon the natural biochemistry; vaccines would not be as, objectionable and would less likely violate people's religion. Many people's religion brings them to ask, would GOD want vaccines to have unnatural to human biology chemicals that will enter a child's sacred blood? Or, would GOD want you to only consider vaccination if it is a SAFER vaccine that does not cause abnormal to the body reactions? Vaccination compliance would increase if vaccines were SAFER vaccines. There would be less violation of one's religion if vaccines were SAFER; without alien, unnatural to human biology chemicals. People believe that GOD does not want His children to be injected with vaccines containing harmful or toxic or unnatural to human biology chemicals! The charity SAFER Vaccines urges you to consider vaccination if it is not against your religion; and if you do consider vaccinating; demand a SAFER vaccine for injection into your child's vital biochemistry! You may be forced to proclaim and obtain your Religious Exemption, it is your stepping stone toward Religious Freedom; so, do perfect it, if necessary! Tell your religious examiner that it is not so, much a matter of how big your faith is; it is much more a matter of how big your GOD is! You merely, must have faith in GOD; for it is

GOD that is doing the mountain moving; and it is GOD who is safeguarding health, through your faith!

I wonder what your religious beliefs or convictions are or what your principles might be. If a chemicalization of unhealthy chemicals were about to befall a child or if some corporate entity was manipulating the world's natural environment with genetic mutations and for the first time in history actually owned life, by owning genetically engineered, mutated seeds; would you be proactive to prevent it or pray that God intervenes to protect the child's chemistry and/ or God's (nature's) authentic/real world? Prayers are always right but please consider personally assisting in doing God's work here and now, on earth. Your devout belief in God means you should be proactive for good and act to protect children and act to protect God's natural world and/or way of life. Take initiative to strike out against corruption or what is unholy; if necessary, use the legal court system in order to aide in God's plan. Do your part to correct what is wrong and help conform to what is good and pure; what God wants and under God's law. Do not be silent or acquiesce or stand idle when something is not right. If you think blood is sacred or agree that parents' have a God given Right to protect their children from unwanted chemicalization of the blood; then act to correct this perversion of the natural order. We need to do all we can to preserve the natural order, so, try and do your part and do your best.

Whatever, your religion or guiding principles are; you and I are very likely in agreement that life must never be owned such as, how the company Monsantos' does now own life in the form of seeds or how the masses of children are enslaved to undergo vaccine chemicalizations. Moreover, there must be no enslavement and/or enforcement of any healthcare; no mandated or enforced vaccine chemicalizations. Vaccine/Drug Company profiteering must not come before securing the safety of our children's internal chemistries and parents must be free to do their very best to keep their children's blood as naturally pure, as possible. The TWO STEPS OF CORRECTION are vital to the unified commitment that it is better to be free than not free in considering what chemicals might be injected. The requirement to obtain parental permission to inject vaccines into your children's delicate and sensitive blood chemistries is basic to freedom. The ability to refuse vaccination based upon religion or religious belief is also, basic to freedom.

Remember, if you have a mustard seed of faith, it is enough to uproot a tall tree. The slightest belief that GOD is with you, protecting you and will see you through whatever trouble you face is all you need; it is not a matter of how big your faith is, it is a matter of how big your GOD is. The inquisition that is demanding of you to confess your faith or tell them what it is in your religious belief that forbids you to allow vaccination is an atrocity of justice and a most vile and egregious violation of Religious Liberty. However, wrong it is, tell them you consider it a blessing that they will listen to you on why vaccination is against GOD's Law or way of life. Turn the other cheek; let them do what they must to allow for you a Religious Exemption and not be made to violate your religion or be enforced to defile your children's clean, sacred blood. Jesus said, "I am the way, the truth and the light and no one comes to the Father except through me."

Have confidence and faith in the power of the LORD; there is no need to be anxious or troubled if you walk with GOD. Faith is present day confidence of a future reality so, if you have faith that your children will not fall victim to an evil, whether in the form of childhood disease or a childhood vaccine chemicalization of unnatural to human biology chemicals, your children will be protected by the power of almighty GOD. When we walk in the light of GOD and have the peace of GOD in our lives we are protected; we can hold our ground and overcome any assault or attempted battery by our enemy. Philippians 4:6-7, "Do not be anxious about anything, but in every situation, by prayer and petition, with thanksgiving, present your requests to GOD. And the peace of GOD, which transcends all understanding, will guard your hearts and your minds in Christ Jesus." Petition GOD for your children's health with all your heart and know they are safe. Isaiah 41:10, "So do not fear, for I am with you; do not be dismayed, for I am your GOD. I will strengthen you and help you; I will uphold you with my righteous right hand."

In seeking Religious Exemption, have the scriptures at hand if the Word of the LORD coincides with your religious belief; memorize the ones you think will make those whom are questioning your religious conviction not to suffer your children with unwanted vaccine chemicalizations so, they are given the Light of GOD and are taught what your religion is. This is not a time to be silent; it is a time to bestow the Truth, the Spirit and the Word of GOD upon them. GOD will always be there to hear and help you. Psalm 4:1-3, "Answer me when I call to you, my righteous GOD. Give me relief from my distress; have mercy on me and hear my prayer. How long will you people turn my glory into shame? How long will love delusions and seek false gods? Know that the Lord has set apart his faithful servant for himself; the Lord hears when I call to him." Pray to GOD constantly, throw yourself at His feet and ask with thankfulness that your children will not be injured by childhood disease and perhaps more importantly, will not be diagnosed with Autism or made to suffer enforced child abuse by mandated vaccination.

If you think it wicked that parents are enforced by vaccination mandate to submit their children to suffer unwanted vaccine chemicalization of unnatural to human biology chemicals and/or that to inject such, alien chemicals to one's natural biochemistry is against GOD's Law then you very likely have a Religious Conviction against vaccination. Psalms 1:1, "Blessed is the one who does not walk in step with the wicked...." So, if you know it true that for a parent to be enforced to suffer their children with chemical vaccine injections is wicked and/or that children have been proven injured by the so called, "Vaccination Court" and despite the fact, of proven vaccine induced injuries that parents must submit by mandated vaccination law their children and it is in your heart that it is wicked to do so, then you are a "blessed one" for not following the false law which requires vaccination or that you refuse to allow vaccination and thereby, do not "walk in step with the wicked". Stand strong in your religious belief; stand strong against evil injections!

Religious Exemption from Vaccinations.

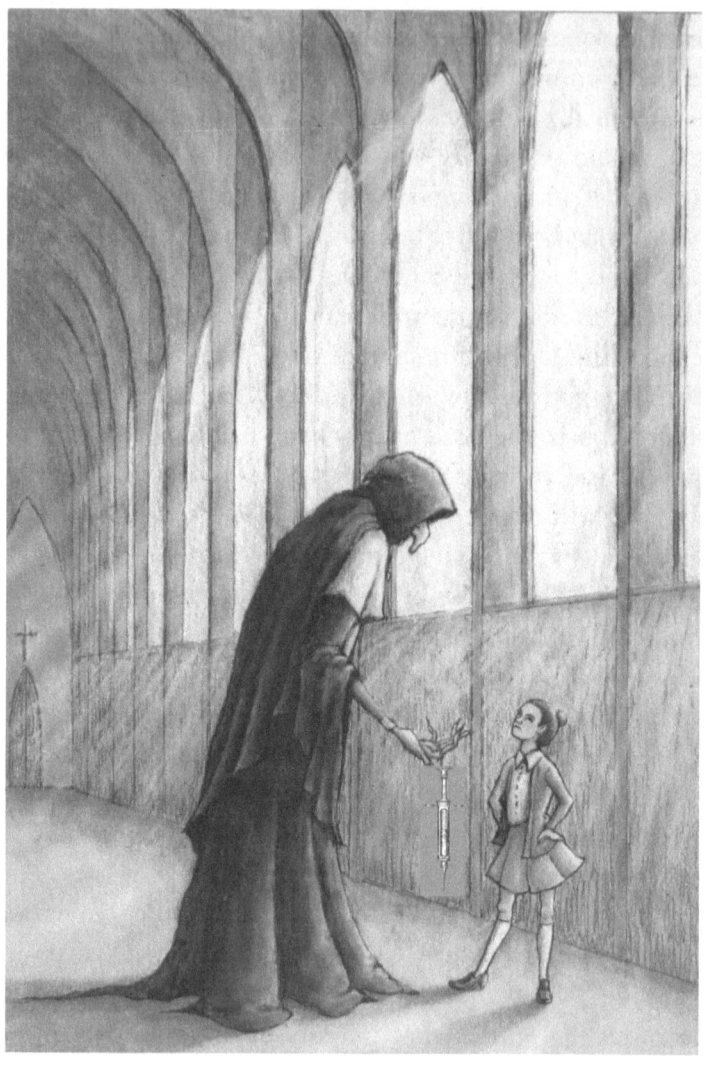

The Constitutional Right of FREEDOM
OF RELIGION protects you from
suffering an unwanted, unnatural to human
biology vaccine chemicalization,
if it violates your religious belief or prevents
the FREE exercise of your
religion. STAND STRONG against what violates your religion!

The bible has multiple passages about healings and health. Mark 6:13, "...and anointed many sick people with oil and healed them." There is an entire health and healing culture whom rely upon essential oils, chiropractic, nutrition, homeopathy, naturopaths and acupuncture etc. instead of drugs, vaccines and surgery. Your religious belief might be that all you need is GOD to be healthy. James 5:14-16, "Is anyone among you sick? Let them call the elders of the church to pray over them and anoint them with oil in the name of the Lord. And the prayer offered in faith will make the sick person well; the Lord will raise them up. If they have sinned, they will be forgiven. Therefore, confess your sins to each other and pray for each other so that you may be healed. The prayer of a righteous person is powerful and effective." Freedom of religion permits you to do the above and to strictly rely and the wisdom of GOD for your health needs without interference or infraction from medical intervention legal mandates or for-profit vaccination that is mandated. GOD wants people to gather in prayer to heal and use natures oils to heal.

If it is with your religion you might state, "I have a religious conviction against vaccination because it violates GOD's design and will. We are made through and by GOD and in His perfect image. Vaccination violates GOD's Will because it forces or stimulates an immune response and/or hijacks GOD's design to do a manmade induced response that is not GOD's design and/or is outside of GOD's natural realm of protection. A hijacked or man induced vaccination immune response can have negative impact on GOD's design. In addition, the fact, that vaccines have been found to be laced with unnatural to GOD's design or unnatural to human biology chemicals it is a further violation of GOD's design or LAW. GOD design for optimum health does not utilize or require chemicals that are not part of what is not in the Image of GOD or is not needed in the normal functioning of a healthy person or developing baby or child. My religion does not tolerate the reliance of drugs or vaccines for my perfectly healthy, perfected by GOD child. My religion forbids the voluntary piercing of the skin by syringe needle and/or the injection of vaccine chemicalizations." GOD is perfect whereas, modern medicine fraught with imperfection.

How many people have been turned into walking zombies from drugs and/or unhealthy chemicalizations? How many iatrogenic (physician induced) injuries or health problems are occurring? Look at how many negative to health or adverse side-effects can occur form taking any drug on the market. Learn how many deaths occur from prescribed medication and how many people become addicted to drugs (walking zombies). There are too many times when medical intervention causes negative health consequences or is unnecessarily performed; when natural healthcare could have been utilized. There are chemicals in vaccines that should not be injected into a tiny baby, little infant or small child. Vaccines can and should be much safer and that is a primary mission of the charity SAFER Vaccines. How many health problems can be helped without the use of medical intervention? Perhaps prayer and/or asking for GOD's help or blessing for health would make a world of difference or a universe of difference. We certainly, should be FREE to pursue our health needs strictly, through the Word of GOD. Our great nation is founded upon religious liberty and within that fundamental liberty Religious Exemption from Vaccination must be freely afforded those whom have the religious belief that does not allow for vaccination.

Freedom of religion is essential for children's well-being and secures GOD's plan for our nation's bright future. Lawmaking buildings and schools must allow for religious freedom and allow religious reminders on its walls. Praying in schools or in our lawmaking buildings must not be against the rules. "ONE NATION UNDER GOD" or reciting the Lord's scripture does not violate the Bill of Rights in fact; it preserves it. We must protect the Constitution, our Right to protect our very own children from unwanted injections of chemicalizations and our "first liberty" freedom of Religion by ending enforced vaccination and allowing unfettered Religious Exemption from vaccination. Praying aloud or saying GOD's name in public places must not be prohibited. There must be liberty to study the TEN COMMANDMENTS and THE WORD OF GOD must reach the crowds. Teach the Word of GOD, right from wrong, good from bad, keep the natural order of things and it will prevent evil. Be FREE to act to prevent chemicalization and not be enslaved to be chemicalized. Live in amazement of the sacred perfection of the world. Thank GOD who delivers you through Jesus Christ our Lord and be FREE to live your life according to the Spirit. May the saving grace of GOD keep you safe and Perfecting Religious Exemption from unwanted vaccine chemicalization injections be your armor of GOD. Put on your armor of GOD to protect your family and secure Freedom of Religion; perfect Religious Exemption from unwanted vaccination. Allow me to give another Religious Exemption scenario that has some important key elements. If I were to find myself at the mercy of a board or group that thinks they are somehow empowered to challenge my faith or my religious sincerity or investigate my religion to see if it merits allowing for a Religious Exemption from vaccination, I would reveal, state and/or preach the following: "If you think you can investigate or question me about my personal relationship with my GOD, you are mistaken however, I will nonetheless take the opportunity to enlighten you. Let me give you a high definition understanding of how my relationship with GOD forbids vaccination. I love GOD first, above anyone and everything. I have been given spiritual insight that there is a New GOD given Commandment for the modern times in which we live. The New Commandment is that as, a parent I shall not with knowledge or out of complacent ignorance pierce my perfectly healthy baby's or child's skin with a vaccine syringe needle and/or inject unnatural to human biology chemicals; I must not imperfect or render impure the sacred blood; it is a sin to desecrate, manipulate or distort the natural and/or GOD given blood chemistry. For to do so, violates GOD's law and is therefore, a sin and can cause unhealthy consequences. Although, I do have knowledge that vaccinations can cause health problems or that vaccines do contain unnatural to human biology chemicals, it is my Religious conviction not to be defiled by vaccine chemicalization injection that is protected by the Constitution under Freedom of Religion that brings me to remonstrate with you to grant my Perfected Religious Exemption from Vaccination. Please, do not force me to sin or abandon my GOD by not granting me a valid Religious Exemption from vaccination.

I would like to end this chapter with a prayer that I was inspired to write that is a basis to LIVE and HEAL by titled, **ABC** Prayer.

ABC PRAYER

HOLY FATHER

Allow the healing of those in need and to heal ourselves
Be always within us, in all we feel, hear and see
Forgive us for our sins, faults and weakness
Protect and guide us in all that we do
Help us to be righteous and strong
Creator of all that is and shall be
Place us on the paths of purity
Heal our bodies and minds
Bring forth all goodness
Shine grace upon us
Purify our souls
Lift our spirits
Enlighten us
Protect us
Bless us
Bestow peace and serenity
Help us to love one another more
Show the way to become one with GOD
The power of GOD is now healing and protecting us
Bless us with **A**bundant Happiness
Bless us with **B**rilliant Health
Bless us with **C**onstant love

AMEN

PREVENTING AUTISM FROM CHEMICALIZATION

This might convince you to become religious about health. The negative to health consequences of injecting babies or children with unnatural to human biology chemicals is immeasurable as the sands on the seashore. The unnatural to human biology chemicals that you are exposed to especially, if injected with, are stumbling stones of health; not stepping stones to health. Chemicals dictate health or Autism! Keep the blood natural or chemically devoid of unnatural to human biology chemicals and health is highly probable; Autism is not. "DIAGNOSIS AUTISM" is being heard at epidemic proportion, it rocks families like an earthquake magnitude infinity and the chemicals in vaccines are a cause in fact, of the Autism epidemic. We need to make vaccination a more intelligent choice! Vaccinating with vaccines that are laced with unnatural to human biology chemicals is not rational; it distorts the vaccine recipients' homogeneous natural biochemistry needed for optimum health. Choose your vaccines wisely; only consider SAFER vaccines! Be uncompromising about one's natural chemical integrity and you will best safeguard against Autism. Distort your biochemistry and abnormal chemical reactions will occur and/or abnormality ensues! Render the blood or biochemistry abnormal; expect abnormality! Autism is mainly caused by abnormalizing the biochemistry. It is of monumental importance to protect your children from abnormal chemicalization. We need the option of the benefits that vaccination can offer however, let us GET THE BAD CHEMICALS OUT of vaccines to make vaccines SAFER (healthier) and thereby, choosing to vaccinate becomes fundamentally rational and no longer is child abuse by abnormal to the body CHEMICALIZATION. Liberty to refuse vaccination based on religious belief is essential to the Constitution and safety.

SAFER vaccines .ORG and .COM are the websites of the charity SAFER vaccines, where you can find out what vaccines are SAFER and learn what vaccines are unsafe due to being laced with anti-health agents or having unnatural to human biology chemicals. The charity and its web sites are designed so that you become educated about health and vaccines. The goal is to prevent you from ever hearing "DIAGNOSIS AUTISM". Do not think that you can inject your tiny baby, small infant or child with vaccines that are laced with unnatural to human biology chemicals and it not cause abnormal reactions within. ABNORMAL REACTIONS = ABNORMALITY! GET THE CHEMICALS OUT of vaccines and you do what is needed to help PREVENT AUTISM. There must be unification to stop vaccine producers from putting chemicals for profit in vaccines. Those who dictate children must endure vaccines that are laced with unnatural to human biology chemicalization do a grave disservice to the welfare of children! There is a bodacious amount of evidence that unnatural to human biology chemicals are wreaking havoc with people's health; we must not inject such, chemicals into babies or children. Vaccines that harbor unnatural to human biology chemicals make the benefit or value of vaccination utterly meaningless.

There can be, should and must be agenda that assures both the optimum health of our children but also, that what ever drug or vaccine is being administered must rightfully pass the parental need and requirement that it has no unnecessary harmful capacity to the optimum health of their children and that parents can by self-preservation right of their children say "NO" to what parents deem not in their children's best interest or is not what is best for their children and/or could be unhealthy for their children. Guarding against unnatural to human biology chemicals is what parents owe to their children's welfare. To inject such chemicalization is an abuse on many levels.

The term "chemicalization" is a word that I coined; the word is readily understood as, describing chemicals entering or infiltrating the body at or after exposure to chemicals. A healthy chemicalization is one that is beneficial to health or needed to be healthy such as, vitamins and minerals; involving chemicals that are building blocks of health that are used by the body to make proteins, enzymes and other metabolic requirements of health. An unhealthy chemicalization is one that is not part of the normal biochemistry, not used by the body as a building block for health instead, it stresses the body, is a burden to the body and/or distorts the normal biochemistry and can interfere with needed normal bioreactions or bioproduction, it can cause abnormal to the body reactions which spawns abnormality; chemicals that are unnatural to human biology that enter the body is an unhealthy chemicalization. Vaccines that have unnatural to human biology chemicals are unhealthy chemicaliztions whereas, SAFER vaccines are not!

Parents are usually always vigilant to safeguard their children, to keep them out of harm's way. There are chemicals that you would not allow your children to eat and the saying, "what you eat you are" puts it nicely how parents are vigilant to not befall their children with bad food chemicalization. Times this valid concern about protecting children from the negative effects of chemicals by a monumental amount when it comes to chemicals which might be injected. There is a temptation to protect your children with vaccination even though it is laced with unnatural to human biology chemicals; avoid this temptation and vaccinate only with SAFER vaccines. Do not abandon what you know to be true; chemicals that are unnatural to human biology should never be injected. If you choose not to control your child's vital chemistry how will you control or assure their biochemical reactions and health? An unsafe vaccine is comparable to a chemical rattle snake—an unhealthy thing to avoid immediately when seen, heard or known of. Why visit your children with a chemicalization danger or throw the chemical dice? Chemicals dictate reactions; health is completely dependent upon proper reactions and the avoidance of abnormal reactions. Unnatural to human biology chemicalization causes abnormal reactions; that equals abnormality.

CHEMICALIZATION AUTISM is the diagnosis and vaccine chemicalization is the main cause! Chemicalization Autism is a diagnosis signifying the cause of the Autism is chemicalization. The Autism epidemic is mainly a chemicalization manifestation due to vaccination. Today expectant mothers and young children are being exposed to more chemicals than ever before. This increased chemical exposure makes it that more imperative that we safeguard against chemicals especially, the chemicals in vaccines. Injection of chemicals into the delicate blood and systems of children is the worst type of exposure because it quickly circulates in the blood unabated and penetrates through the blood brain barrier to penetrate the brain; doping the brain cells with whatever unnatural to the biology chemicals that are in the vaccine. Children are more susceptible than ever before to injected chemicals because they are more frequently exposed to unnatural to human biology chemicals than ever before from the environment, clothing and tainted foods and therefore, one's chemical tolerance can be challenged or maxed out prior to vaccine CHEMICALIZATION. However, make no mistake, Autism is mainly caused by the abnormal to the body chemicals of vaccines; Autism can be an injection away! The TWO STEPS OF CORRECTION stated in my book, SAFER *vaccines*, SAFER *CHILDREN* and reiterated in this book, PREVENTING AUTISM will assure SAFER vaccines with no bad for health chemicals. The rate of Autism will rage on until the TWO STEPS are implemented.

Everyone has a chemicalization breaking point where being infiltrated with unnatural to human biology chemicals causes health to degenerate. How many non-consented to shots is intolerable depends upon your tolerance for chemical abuse. Your breaking point to no longer blindly obey the erroneous vaccination mandate can depend on if you know someone whose health has been devastated by vaccine chemical injections. It has become much too common to personally know of someone claiming that vaccinations are the cause of their children's Autism; it is an epidemic! Parents know best when their children are injured by vaccinations. **Diagnosis Autism** is what is being told to multitudes of parents after they submit children for vaccinations and they contemporaneously observe their children's health disintegrate into **AUTISM**. Preventing chemical exposure is possibly the most important health protection; parents must be **FREE TO PROTECT children from vaccine anti-health chemicals**. Vaccine producers and those who advocate injecting children with unclean vaccines that have chemicals for strictly profit and not safety; need to learn the lesson of the difference between a laboratory and a lavatory and thereby, stop putting crap in our children's vaccines. We want the safest vaccines possible and no rational person can argue otherwise and only the reckless would allow the chemicals that have been found in vaccines to be in or remain in vaccines. It is staggering at any level that vaccine producers would purposely put certain chemicals in vaccines such as, but not limited to thimerosal (a mercury derivative) or aluminum and thereby throw our children under the bus. **Children desperately deserve and need SAFER vaccines that do not compromise their vital to health biochemistry. TWO STEPS OF CORRECTION are needed to assure SAFER vaccines!**

It is difficult to calculate all the negative to health impact from **injecting babies with abnormal to their body or unnatural to their normal biochemistry particulates found in vaccines, however, know the egregious injections of multiple chemicalizations are harmful. Parents of children diagnosed with Autism are wise to prevent a progressive or more severe Autism by not chemically compromising the children any further so, consider to never ever again inject them with any vaccine that has any degree of unnatural to human biology chemicals.** Children with Autism need their parents to protect them by doing everything they can to rid their children of harmful chemicals and assure that they are not ever again infiltrated by unnatural to the body chemicals. In addition, make their physically and emotionally environments health promoting. Diet should be pure with no harmful chemicals and be charged with the vitamins, minerals and live enzymes which are necessary to promote optimum health. Create an atmosphere for Autistic children of constant affection, love, caring and nurturing. Visualizations and perceptions should strive to become very positive and health promoting. The next chapter entitled, "**POSITIVE HEALTH MEASURES**" gives more insight on helping Autistic children live a near normal life and recover from being chemically compromised.

All the natural and non-invasive methods of healthcare and healing should be freely sought to improve the health of the Autistic child; one should not be handcuffed to rely or robotically take drugs that chemically compromise you. Taking drug chemicals for every little thing that is wrong is very unwise and children suffering from chemicalization Autism should not be further chemically compromised with drugs that have too long a list of negative to health effects! To make rules or law that people must submit their perfectly healthy children for chemical injections is undemocratic, totalitarian, tyrannical and CHILD ABUSE BY CHEMICALIZATION. Be FREE to do everything you can to protect your children and have the liberty to create a health promoting natural environment for your children and once obtained, preserve it; without governmental interference or commands. To be enforced to chemicalize children with unnatural to human biology chemicals is far beyond unreasonable; it is nothing less than insanity and is tyrannical medical intervention child abuse. Basic liberty requires PARENTS TO BE IN SUPREME control over their children's welfare! What will serve best to assure vaccine safety and prevent children from exposure to bad chemicals or unsafe vaccines is for parents to be FREE to refuse any vaccine that they think is not chemically safe; there must be LIBERTY TO REJECT INJECTIONS! History has shown that vaccines have chemicals that are extremely, objectionable.

You need to protect your children from UNNATURAL TO HUMAN BIOLOGY CHEMICALS and your children desperately need your protection! A key to health is not to toxify and to detoxify if you have been exposed to unnatural to human biology chemicals. We all now, know that certain unnatural to human biology chemicals cause cancer; we too slowly are learning that the INJECTION of unnatural too human biology chemicals causes abnormal reactions and abnormal reactions equals, abnormality. Those that first recognize the truth or that first state new knowledge or wisdom are usually condemned and censored. Those that came up with the world is flat or that the world is not the center of the universe or that it is not the sun which revolves around the earth but rather, the earth that revolves around the sun, all were initially condemned and censored. What is established or ingrained into our minds as good or beneficial makes new beneficial knowledge harder to surface and difficult to be recognized; and the indoctrination into vaccination is safe, is the epitome of this difficulty. Vaccines can and must be made safer! Vaccines should not have unnatural to human biology chemicals since, it obviously, will be injected into developing tiny babies. Too many advocates of vaccines do not want people questioning vaccine safety or content; they condemn anyone that dare seek to achieve SAFER vaccines. This belligerent attitude does not allow for possible improvement in vaccine safety; it is dangerous and is not in the best interest of children's welfare.

Vaccine makers' posture that vaccines are safe enough but, try telling that to the parents who are crying their eyes out when their children are needlessly injured by an injected vaccine chemicalization. There is always room for improvement in healthcare especially, for vaccines that have been found to have such, chemicals. Certain chemicals in vaccines are adjuvants; it makes the vaccine work better. Adjuvants may be considered needed but, it may be too dangerous and there may be safer alternatives; and when it comes to chemicalization less is better than more. There are preservatives in vaccines that need to be analyzed for safety or harmful propensities. There are chemicals in vaccines that are more for profiteering than for children's safety. We are being exposed to all kinds of harmful chemicals among the worst are from plastics but, by far, the most common unhealthiest chemicalization exposure for babies is from being injected with vaccines laced with unnatural to human biology chemicals. It is therefore, a state of emergency that we render SAFER vaccines for all our children! In the United States, local and state governments are banning the sale of baby bottles (plastic lined) that contain the chemical bisphenol A (BPA); let us, wisely ban vaccines that are laced with unnatural to human biology chemicals. Even as, a precautionary principle, it is wise to ban vaccines having chemicals which derange, upset, alter, manipulate or distort the natural biochemistry. What disrupts the normal biochemistry should not be in vaccines; it needs to be removed, under a precautionary principle! Do not throw anti-health chemicalization dice!

To chemically compromise your children by injection is not what parents bargained for when they innocently bring their children in to be vaccinated. There must be full and complete disclosure of all the chemicals in vaccines and parents must have the fundamental liberty to refuse a vaccine if they determine it is not in their children's best interest. Parents' MUST NOT acquiesce in being left no choice but to submit their children for unwanted chemical injections. It is in the best interest of children that vaccinations be based upon parental consent and input. Vaccinations must no longer be permitted to intrude upon the parental obligation and responsibility of caring for and/or safeguarding their children. The level of violation to parental Rights is off the scale; the injustice too extreme, and the results are horrific. Children are being injured because parents are not given their fundamental Right to refuse unwanted vaccine chemicalizations and do to the injustice that producers of vaccines cannot be litigated against for vaccine induced injuries. It is a perversion of caring for children to enforce inject babies with chemicals. I recommend vaccinating but, only with what you are sure is a SAFER vaccine!

Nowhere, in healthcare is medical intervention enforced upon the public as is done with vaccinations; it wrongfully, oppressively and unjustifiably is enforced. These are perfectly healthy children that are being enforced to be injected and chemically compromised. Even if vaccines had no history of adverse reactions or that it was not a fact, that almost a billion dollars have been paid to the vaccine injured after being proven that the vaccine caused injury by the Vaccination Court; the decision to vaccinate should squarely rest with parents as, is all other healthcare decisions for children. The long reach of the profiteering pharmaceutical industry has manipulated a sure way to permanently, make mega-profits. Big government has been overwhelmingly lobbied to make these unjust mandated vaccination laws that assure the mega-profiteering from an enforced vaccination ENSLAVED public. Children are in desperate need of their parents informed consent/DENIAL protection therefore, INFORMED DENIAL/informed consent law must control vaccinations just as, it applies to all types and modes of medical interventions. Those who are responsible for exposing our children to the harm of unnatural to the body chemicals such as, but not limited to thimerosal and aluminum or that callously enforce it upon children through a mal-vaccination mandate, HAVE NO SHAME, THEY DON'T KNOW HOW TO BLUSH. They have even made it so, that if your child is injured from injected vaccine chemicalization you cannot even hold the vaccine maker' accountable or liable or make it pay! You cannot deny the objective reality of the problems caused by having even the slightest degree of unnatural to human biology chemicals in children's vaccines or the further problem obstructing greater safety and/or negative attitude not to GET THE CHEMICALS OUT or massive complication of not holding vaccine producers accountable and liable when its vaccines do induce injuries.

Please, recognize that vaccination is big business and that Big Pharma lobbies to keep vaccination mandated to assure profiteering. One should question whether so many vaccinations are needed and raise both eyebrows off your face in bewilderment as to, why any vaccination is mandated under a biased profit-based system. Vaccines can and do cause injury so, parents rightfully should make the decision; perfectly healthy children need to have their vaccination decisions made by parents as is, for all other children's healthcare decisions. When it comes to making money it too often causes the need for the medical intervention. Practically all surgeons have an inherent financial conflict of interest 'That's because they are paid approximately ten times more money to perform surgery than to manage your problem conservatively.' —James Rickert, MD, an orthopedic surgeon in Bedford, Indiana. In addition, many times the need for vaccination or a diagnosis is very often erroneous. A patient sent his slides to three different pathologists and got three different answers, 'I got very upset on hearing that. Now I never rely on just one pathology exam. If your doctor finds something, ask him to send your slides to a nationally recognized reference lab—not just one or two slides but the whole lot—and get a second interpretation.'

—Bert Vorstman, MD, a prostate cancer specialist in Coral Springs, Florida. The practice of medicine is far from perfect, there is always room for improvement. There is nothing wrong with confidence but, there is wrong with arrogance. There needs to be a desire for SAFER vaccines, do not succumb to unhealthy chemicalization; we must overcome vaccine safety inadequacy. They must want wisdom to achieve SAFER vaccines; it is a matter of attitude. The TWO STEPS OF CORRECTION is what is needed to prevent needless vaccine induced injury.

It is absolute absurd that parents' supreme Right is being blocked, that they are not enabled to safeguard their children welfare or biochemical integrity. The mandated vaccination law is an enigma to the entire healthcare field; it stands all alone as the only enforced healthcare which eviscerates parents' supreme Right to protect their children from vaccine exposures laced with unnatural to human biology chemicals or is deemed by parents as, too dangerous to inject. The further audacity of vaccination extremists whom do not have an understanding hearing heart to step up to the plate of increasing vaccine safety or heed vaccine consumers' call to improve vaccine safety through the removal of unnatural to the body chemicals from vaccines, fuels parent's complete turnoff to vaccination. We have two ears but, only one mouth so, vaccine producers need to spend more time listening instead of talking; listen to vaccine consumers and merely speak on how great or safe vaccines supposedly are. After all, these are our children and by the highest law parents are FREE to protect their children. BE FREE TO REJECT INJECTIONS!

Law must consistently allow for you to be the very best parents that you aspire to be; there must be no law that denigrates or supersedes parenting. Mandated vaccinations dictate parents to inject their children even when parents think it not in their children's best health interest or is too dangerous to inject. Thank GOD for GOD and Freedom of Religion that is Perfected by Religious Exemption from Vaccination.

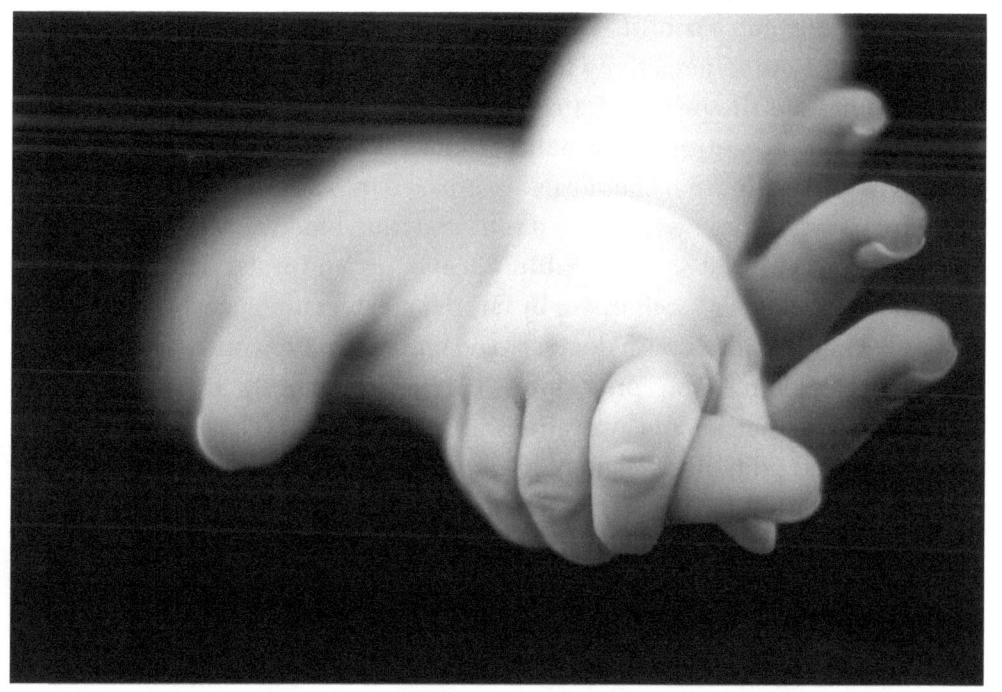

YOUR CHILDREN RELY ON YOU TO PROTECT THEM FROM UNHEALTHY, UNNATURAL TO HUMAN BIOLOGY CHEMICALIZATION.

Chemicalization is the enemy! Chemicals present in the body and blood take part in reactions and have direct impact on bioproduction. Abnormal to human biology chemicals cause abnormal reactions and that makes for ABNORMALITY. Wisdom tells us to safeguard expecting mothers and children from such, chemicalization. An *Environmental Health Perspectives* report published online October 6, drawing on data from 249 mothers and their children in Cincinnati, Ohio, associated prenatal BPA exposure with more aggressive and hyperactive behavior in girls at age 2. There is no question that alien to the body chemicals are destructive to health and is causing abnormality. There was a study that linked BPA exposure to recurrent miscarriage among Japanese women. Think how crazy it is, too conclude that unnatural to human biology chemicals in vaccines which are injected into babies are not harmful. Chemicalization causes health problems ranging from hyperactivity to cancer; chemicalization from unsafe vaccines are the primary cause of the autism epidemic. Preserving health or preventing abnormality is more about what chemicals are in us especially, what chemicals are injected into us rather, than what drugs or vaccines we take! Keep your body and blood chemistry pure and you will best secure health! Cleaner air and water are a must however, cleaner vaccines are by far, the greater emergency!

Many hospitals push doctors to do more operations and pay them more for doing more procedures (conflict of interest). It has been estimated that 25% of operations are unnecessary. The Cleveland Clinic has said, 'this system of paying doctors is so ethically immoral that it started paying its doctors a flat salary no matter how many operations they do.' When it comes to vaccinations doctors are not on the same page in that many think not all are needed and many doctors think that informed consent should rule over vaccinations. Almost all doctors think that SAFER vaccines that have less or no unnatural to human biology chemicals is in the best interest of all children. One of the main reasons why Chiropractors do not have hospital rights is because it prevents back operations and that it helps people recover from aliments without the use of drugs or medical procedures and that means a loss of big money to hospitals. Many doctors and hospitals are ethical; many are not. Your children need your uncompromised, incorruptible, principled decision on vaccinations! If parents control vaccination delivery vaccines will not have chemicals for profit and not safety. The TWO STEPS OF CORRECTION of the charity, SAFER vaccines, will induce SAFER vaccines for children. The priority must be safety; not the mere hollow accomplishment of vaccination compliance!

The Pharmaceutical industry has so many lobbyists pushing politicians around or to turn a blind eye to vaccine safety requirements that nobody is doing anything to assure vaccine safety measures. The US Department of Health and Human Services (HHS) admitted in a federal court stipulation signed on July 6, 2018 that it never submitted biannual reports to Congress detailing improvements in vaccine safety made by HHS as required by the 1986 National Childhood

Vaccine Injury Act (NCVIA) at 42 U.S.C Sec. 300aa-27(c). It is incredulous that there is a total lack of following legal requirements that assure our children's safety. The first report was due in 1989 and was supposed to be followed with reports every two years but, no reports have occurred; not filing required reports indicates no improvements in vaccine safety and not adhering to proving required improvements is the reckless endangerment of our children. The admission was obtained in a lawsuit filed by the Informed Consent Action Network to compel HHS to produce the requested documents (that do not exist). The Informed Consent Action Network was represented by Robert F. Kennedy, Jr. My first book, *STING OF THE MEDICAL MOSQUITO*, was handed to Robert F. Kennedy, Jr. and hopefully it helped energize him into beneficial action. Apparently, the HHS has fallen susceptible to lobbyists and left our children fall victim to less or no vaccine safety quality control. It is no wonder that unnatural to human biology chemicals have been found in vaccines! The evidence is overwhelming that children need their parents to protect them from the lack of protection by those entities charged with protecting the public; no one is better suited or has better reason to assure children's safety than parents thus, parents must BE FREE TO REJECT INJECTIONS that they deem too dangerous to inject and/or have unhealthy chemicals.

Although, the primary cause of Autism is from injecting unhealthy chemicals; we should strive to eliminate all sources of unnatural to the body chemicalization so, not to chemically compromise children. Everything the Autistic child eats, or encounters should be analyzed for its chemical content, to be sure there are no further abnormal to the body chemical exposures. Anti-health chemical agents are the enemy and enemy number one, is vaccine chemicalization; it is the most dangerous of chemicalizations because it is injected. Autism can regress, and optimum health can once again resonate, if no more chemical compromising and/or toxification take place and if detoxification occurs. The main key to the prevention of Autism is to assure pure blood chemistry and the main way to recover from Autism is to regain naturally pure blood chemistry. Prevent exposure to unnatural to the body chemicals and never inject such, chemicals. Anti-health chemicals must not be injected! Once Autism is diagnosed begin purification of the blood. Prevention of unnatural to human biology chemical intake is essential to prevent and recover from Autism; it is in your children's best interest.

Parents should be aware of all the various chemical exposure possibilities and immediately eliminate all exposures that are anti-health chemicalizations. Make no mistake, toxic to the body chemicals cause Autism and the injection of these harmful chemicals is the main etiology of Autism and gateway to all kinds of health issues. There are a few surprising sources of chemical toxic exposures like when independent studies found that 38% of 50 retail milk samples collected in 10 major cities were contaminated with sulfa drugs and antibiotics used to treat sick cattle. Consequently, these chemicals have been ingested by babies, infants and children. Sulfa-methazine has also been found in milk and this chemical is a suspected carcinogen. **Everyone is susceptible to health problems from unnatural to the body chemicals. There are many sources of contamination however, vaccine injected chemicals are the most common cause of a critical chemical mass syndrome that can lead to Autism. Upset your biochemistry and the life generating bio-reactions faulter; ABNORMAL BIOCHEMISTRY = ABNORMALITY! Prevent your children from being chemically compromised and you prevent your children from "DIAGNOSIS AUTISM." Proper parenting requires that you protect your children from harmful chemicalizations; only consider the injection of SAFER vaccines and do make sure it is a SAFER vaccine! Think before you leap into vaccinating with a chemically compromising vaccine. Safeguard your children's vital life-giving blood biochemistry. Be FREE to be the best parents you can be! Think of the consequences of injecting toxic to the body chemicals such as, but not limited to, thimerosal (a mercury derivative and known neurotoxin) and Aluminum, a high magnetic conductor upon the fragile developing systems of your tiny baby, infant or child! To do so, is the reckless endangerment of children and CHILD ABUSE by chemicalization.**

Abnormal to the body or unnatural to human biology chemicalization is infiltrated by our way of life and we are being adversely affected by it. The Autism Epidemic is partially a result of environmental and food toxic chemicalization, but it the main causation are injections of the multiple vaccines with all its alien to the body chemicalizations. There are about 30,000 animal drugs in use today of which their residues can be found in meat, milk and eggs. Many years can elapse between the granting of "emergency" approval to ban veterinary prescription drugs and the end of their use. Use of banned drugs can continue illegally for instance, Chloramphenicol, an antibiotic banned for use in meat animals since 1968 because of its residues can cause a **fatal blood disorder in humans**, continued to be used for over 20 years after it was banned. Hormonal drugs typically are used in animals to promote growth and of course to assure greater profit; these harmful chemicals find their way into our children's meals. In fact, it is common that hormonal pellets are placed in illegal points or in double dosage in animals that are destined to be eaten by our children. Gentian violet an animal drug is a **known carcinogen** and yet it is nevertheless continuing to be used as a mold-inhibiting additive to poultry feed. **There is a long list of drugs that cause cancer in laboratory animals that the FDA still allows for common use.** It is obvious that Drug Companies and/or Vaccine Producers and the FDA do not hold our best interest. **With all these chemical exposures; it is that much more imperative NOT TO INJECT VACCINES WITH UNNATURAL BODY CHEMICALS!** The FDA and **Big Pharma** are biased toward one another and too often bounce back and forth landing golden jobs with each other; the conflict of interest is off the scale. If vaccinations were not so unconscionably profitable there would be NO VACCINATION MANDATES.

They put mercury in vaccines as a preservative to stop spoilage; this toxic chemical for profit assures greater profit because the pharmaceutical rep only comes to the doctor's office rarely instead, of regularly and stock piling of huge sales can take place with no risk of returns from spoilage. Most parents or vaccine recipients would rather, have a vaccine without such, toxic chemical preservatives or choose a vaccine that has salt as a preservative or select a vaccine with a short shelf-life without any preservative or poison. Parents must become proactive to protect their family from bad chemicalization exposures! Exposure to chemicals effectuates disease and Autism. Become informed and acutely aware of the long list of chemicals that can enter your children and take affirmative action to prevent all unnatural chemical infiltrations. The next time someone points a vaccine injection at your children with intension to inject; make absolutely, sure it will not be chemically compromising your children and setting the course for AUTISM! If someone unintelligently remarks or presumes that the chemical exposure is insignificant; think about the overall cumulative chemicalization danger and that because vaccines are directly injected into your children's delicate and susceptible blood, it poses a truly ominous threat. The injection of chemically laced vaccines can tip the chemical scale enough to cause a critical mass chemical syndrome and thereby, SPAWN AUTISM.

The TWO STEPS of CORRECTION will GET THE CHEMICALS OUT of vaccines and stop the prevalence of DIAGNOSIS AUTISM. We must take every measure and precaution to make sure the needle puncturing children's skin is clean and the vaccine to be injected is clean! Make sure the vaccine that is about to become systemic is devoid of ALEIN, UNNATURAL TO THE BODY CHEMICALS. Recognize that the origin of Autism is mainly due to foreign chemical infiltrations and resultant abnormal reactions from their toxic presence and/or propensities. Vaccine producers must no longer exploit and use for their profiteering agenda the Police Power of the State to enforce vaccinate. The Police Power must not be used to guarantee profit from mandated or enforced vaccine sales or be used to place our children's health in chemical peril; it must not assure a vaccination monopoly and/or vaccination mandated profiteering! The perversion and injustice of denying parents their fundamental right of Self-determined healthcare and its basic liberty to refuse the unwanted medical intervention of vaccination must end and SAFER vaccines will concurrently result!

The degree of harm that chemically laced vaccine injections cause makes the violation of the Police Power that much more egregious. There are different injuries that can take place in life, some injuries are minor, taking merely a short period of time to recover and/or heal while other injuries cut deeper and are much more difficult to recover and/or heal. The type or degree of harm that can come from enforced, no choice but to vaccinate, injections can be devastating to health and plaque the chemicalization victim for life. Make no mistake, chemical exposure is the number one enemy of health, the number one cause of health problems and vaccine chemical injections are the most formidable enemy cloaked in sheep's clothing. There does not need to be a tradeoff that one must suffer unnatural to human biology chemicalization in order to have the proposed benefit of vaccination. We may need or want vaccination to prevent childhood disease however; we do not need the chemical exposure risk. **We must rid vaccines of their chemical harms and trust in a strictly voluntary vaccination program.** We also must recognize all sources of chemical exposure and do everything humanly possible to stop it.

The Environmental Protection Agency (EPA) ranked **pesticide residues in food** as the nation's number 3 environmental **cancer risk,** right after toxic chemicals exposure in the work place and radon gas exposure in the home. Yes, chemicals introduced into the body disrupt the normal functioning and biochemistry of the body. **Pesticides are big business just like chemical vaccinations are.** Some pesticides, known as "**systemic pesticides**" spread throughout the plant and just cannot be rinsed or washed off. United States farmers now use approximately 10 times more insecticide than 50 years ago. Children that are raised on farms which have a high frequency of exposures to pesticides and/or herbicides have a **marked increase** in the frequency of **cancers and birth defects.** Chemicals called Neonicotinoids have been banned because it is thought responsible for killing off the Bee population; mass use of chemicals destroy life and mass use of vaccine chemicals destroy health; **spawning AUTISM.** What chemicals do you want circulating throughout your children's bloodstreams? Liberty to self-govern what is or is not allowed to enter your body and blood is essential to self-preservation and to do the same for your children is essential to parenting.

Children throughout America are having their unhealthy fill of chemical exposures. **The chemical exposure base has been increasing over the generations as we become entrenched in a chemical ridden world and when this is combined with the chemical onslaught of chemically laced vaccinations the possibility of a critical mass chemical syndrome increases exponentially. How many chemicals can a human be exposed to until health is placed in jeopardy or until**

x

CHEMICALIZATION AUTISM becomes a reality? How many vaccines of unnatural to human biology chemicalizations can a baby withstand? Perhaps many or perhaps 1 or maybe none! In order, for parents to best protect their children they need to be cognizant of what chemicals their children might be encountering and be vigilant not to expose their children to chemicals that destroy health. An important study that should be performed is to compare the Autism rate among these farm children that have been exposed to a higher degree of chemicals and are also exposed to the enforced vaccinations, as compared, to the general population that does not have the farm related chemical exposures. The farm exposed fully vaccinated group will likely have a higher Autism rate than the general population fully vaccinated group unless the chemical exposure from vaccinations are so significant a cause of Autism that additional source of chemical exposure cannot be detected or register as an additional causation of Autism. If diagnosed with Autism follow the chemical trail to not repeat chemical exposure; it is best to avoid all chemicals that are unnatural to the body and absolutely, avoid further toxic chemical vaccine injections. Become a detective of what caused the health degeneration, seek out the CHEMICAL culprits and you will more than likely discover that vaccinations were the main etiology of Autism. SAVE YOUR CHILDREN FROM AUTISM BT SAVING THEM FROM BAD CHEMICALIZATION! Do not let Autism from Chemicalization become your child's reality.

How many injections of vaccine chemicals in conjunction with all other sources of toxicity that children encounter before a chemical critical mass episode is reached can only be attempted to be quantified. The chemical exposure madness must be stopped at all costs; our children's lives are at stake. The TWO STEPS OF CORRECTION is the giant leap in the right direction to protect children's welfare and is in their best interest. We can no longer stand idle or be expected to endure our children's continual increasing exposures to alien to the body chemicals. The ABOLISHMENT of vaccination SLAVERY is needed to end these chemical exposures and to regain; FREEDOM of SELF-DETERMINED HEALTHCARE and PARENTS' RIGHT TO PROTECT CHILDREN and allow fundamental FAMILY AUTONOMY.

What results from bombarding our bodies with foreign to the body chemicals is an altering of the normal biochemistry that makes for abnormal biological reactions and the prevention of required for health reactions. Consequently, there is now a tremendous amount of people being diagnosed with Dementia and/or Alzheimer's, Cancer, Vision problems, Diabetes and an **AUTISM EPIDEMIC**. All these health problems continue to be increasing despite modern medicine because ONE CANNOT FIGHT A CHEMICALLY INDUCED PROBLEM BY INTYRODUCING MORE CHEMICALS IN THE FORM OF DRUGS AND/OR CHEMICALLY LAIDEN VACCINES. Our bodies are all sensitive to unnatural to the body chemical exposure and we all have tolerance levels that once reached cause our neurological and endocrine systems to malfunction. **Chemical infiltration is the key causation of most of today's health problems. PREVENT CHEMICALIZATION AND YOU PREVENT MOST HEALTH PROBLEMS!** Government must not mandate vaccine injections especially injections of any degree of unhealthy chemicals. We must be FREE to self-control what runs throughout our bodies! Be FREE to decide as our children's parents, what is best for our children!

If one is not exposed to harmful chemicals, one has a much greater chance at being healthy and not need to go to the doctor. Compare the quickly growing population of those who have claimed a religious exemption so not to be vaccinated or those that home school to remain unvaccinated to that of the vaccinated population; the numbers of those with Autism reveal that vaccine chemicals are the main etiology of Autism. In addition, compare the unvaccinated with the vaccinated as to, how often the children have had to run to the doctors or have been on antibiotics or had fevers, asthma, petite mal seizures, convulsions, headaches, allergies, skin rashes and missed school days. You will find that the comparison is startling; making it obvious that the injecting of vaccine chemicals, after vaccine chemicals, after vaccine chemicals; are the main etiology of most children's health problems. You must be FREE to protect your children from vaccine chemicalizations and have your healthy, unvaccinated children, enter school; unmolested or prejudiced! VACCINATION SLAVERY' ENFORCES CHEMICALIZATION CHILD ABUSE! Vaccine producers act with impunity when its vaccines contain unnatural to human biology chemicals and/or induce harm, making the vaccination mandate even more egregious.

Obviously, the laws of chemistry apply to the chemicals inside of our bodies. When you pollute your sensitive internal chemistry; renegade reactions are induced and many of the normal, essential for health reactions are blocked. When a child is suspected of becoming Autistic because of vaccination and parents do not let their other children be vaccinated because of it; a very revealing statistic occurs. What is revealed is that the siblings of the child that was rendered Autistic do not become Autistic; their **health remains intact because they were not vaccinated**. The fact, that siblings with practically the same genetic makeup are or are not Autistic and the only eye-opening variable is vaccination strongly points to vaccine chemicalization as the cause in fact, of Autism. The genetic causation is proven wrong; the main cause of the child's Autism is that the child was chemically compromised by the vaccine chemicalization. One cannot expect to remain 100% normal and/or optimally healthy when injected with foreign to the body, chemically laced vaccines. **Keep clear of chemical exposure and you will not cause health problems. Make vaccine producers clean-up their vaccines and the main reason for the Autism epidemic will cease. Parents must be FREE to keep their children's blood pure!**

When the natural range of chemicals are circulating in the blood and feeding the brain and body cells optimum health is possible and highly probable; the normal biochemistry allows for the normal physiology and/or needed biological function. When this natural chemistry range is thrown out of kilter or rendered abnormal by the infiltration of injected anti-health chemicals then the health homeostasis is disrupted, and AUTISM can be spawned. You cannot chemically adulterate children's blood WITH BAD VACCINE CHEMICALS at such an alarming vaccination schedule and expect children to remain healthy; its illogical. To enforce injections of vaccine chemical insults that alter the normal chemical integrity is a breach of the trust that we have placed in vaccine producers and its puppet government. Parents are well-advised to trust in the laws of chemistry and not in the erroneous vaccination mandate laws. Protect your children's chemistry; keep it natural and pure! Parents' must be FREE to safeguard their children's natural chemical geometry!

One example of just **how chemically and/or molecular sensitive we are** and the health problems that occur due to the slightest change to our internal chemistry is seizures that can occur in a Diabetic patient. When insulin levels and/or sugar levels become abnormal a seizure can occur. Interestingly, the changes are so slight that modern medicine has a difficult time detecting the changes UNTIL A SEIZURE IS APPARENT. VACCINE CHEMICALIZATION EFFECTS AND/OR THEIR AFFECTS UPON THE VACCINATION RECIPIENT ARE OFTEN UNDETECTED UNTIL, A FULL-BLOWN AUTISM DIAGNOSIS IS RENDERED. Look at the signs and symptomology of the Autistic such as, the neurological malfunction or abnormality and realize that when these signs and symptoms first appeared they insidiously began until a full-blown Autism was spawned or another unfortunate vaccine chemicalization of unnatural to human biology chemicals was inoculated. Observing parents have reported that they detected something wrong or was beginning to go wrong or felt or detected the abnormal chemical changes that caused abnormality or unhealth in their children at the time or proximate to a vaccine chemicalization was injected into their child. Parents have a special sense or bond with their offspring that alerts them to their children's needs and cautions parents when a harm is threatening or an evil is lurking.

In seizures, the subtle body chemical changes can be detected by man's best friend, the dog; dogs can actually warn us to act to either normalize sugar levels and/or insulin levels long before the chemical problem escalates into a terrible seizure. Dog's sense of smell gives them the capability to detect the chemical changes in the person who is heading toward a seizure. What this shows us is that **our health is very dependent upon a stable natural chemistry and that the slightest deviation can cause problems and that the chemical alterations that cause abnormality can be detected by dogs and/or felt by parents. Abnormal chemical occurrence or unhealthy chemicalization's** effects or affects have a geometric register that is observable and/or detectable! Vaccines' unnatural to human biology chemicals that are injected into the blood and/or body is a **definite chemical deviation** from the norm. Perhaps dogs can be trained to detect the chemical changes and/or chemical chaos that ensue after alien vaccine chemicals are injected and/or as Autism begins or before full blown Autism occurs. Dog's acute sense of smell or their ability to detect magnetic field or energy changes can be used to alert us to health degeneration subtle health facts before parents hear **"DIAGNOSIS AUTISM"**.

Someday soon, dogs will be used for early detection of all kinds of health problems that most humans are incapable or not in tune to detect such as, depression, Cancer or Autism. Dogs have become an extension of ourselves, they can detect things that we cannot and then communicate the alarming fact to us. The spiraling chemical reactive chaos form chemically laced vaccines be told. Dogs that undergo a bad vaccination also, often are dealt health problems. Dogs often exhibit excessive licking at the vaccination site and uncontrollable hyperactivity for long periods of time and on occasion develop permanent trembling, digestive disorders and other health issues. **The universal laws of chemistry apply to all life; so, keep your children's biochemistry pure and/or natural and then abnormal reactions and/or abnormality becomes remote! Inject SAFER vaccines to keep the biochemistry pure as, possible. Visit the web-site SAFERvaccines .ORG or .COM for SAFER vaccines knowledge. There is no controlling reason why you cannot consider SAFER vaccines!**

One more revealing bark about man's best friend, all dogs originated from wild, wolfs or coyotes or foxes, that all have a genetic wild, very vicious propensity. Selective breeding and **changing the animals ENVIORNMENT has changed the genetic expression** of the now, approximate 400 different species of dogs that man has had their hand in creating; **to be genetically coded docile** and man's best friend. Dogs can be changed back to their ancestry vicious propensity by doing the opposite. Analogously, the creation of a certain negative to health environment triggers our genes to help cause health problems such as, but not limited to Autism. Changing back to a natural chemical environment should over time allow natural, healthy and/or normal, life force once again and therefore end the increasing Autism epidemic. Every 7 years almost all our cells are replaced thus, given time one could become healthy. We must **GET THE CHEMICALS OUT** of our children and/or **OUT OF THE VACCINES** that we inject into them!

There was an experiment in Russia, attempting to take the aggressive nature out of wild foxes; it took only 8 generations of selective breeding of allowing only the calmest foxes to breed and a regular nurturing, petting environment, with humans to render the fox genetically domestic and no longer aggressive. What this all points out is that our genes can be turned on or off according to the environment that we are in and perceive. Keeping our natural environment that promotes health and happiness is Nature's lesson. **Generations of the vaccinated**, with alien, unnatural to the body chemicals can alter cellular and the gene's environment, will likely cause a mutation, an altered state or changed genetic propensities and/or a **hereditary form of AUTISM**. Diagnosis Autism is from chemically changing the cellular environment and can turn hereditary.

We have been living under the tyranny of enforced vaccination suffering our perfectly healthy children with unnatural to human biology chemicalization by injection with no viable liberty to refuse the vaccination even when the parents are either not convinced of the vaccines safety or are convinced that the vaccine is not safe and/or is too dangerous to inject! Parents have a GOD given supreme Right to care for their children and under this most fundamental and all-important of Rights parents must be completely FREE to decide if a vaccine is or is not in their children's best interest. Parental protection of their offspring from what parents deem is a too dangerous vaccine injection is an invaluable, unalienable Right that cannot legally be taken or diminished or even temporarily shelved. The mandate of vaccination especially, in perpetuity is therefore, illegal and must be stricken down for being so! Vaccines have become too dangerous, being proven to have unnatural to human biology chemicals and have induced or caused many injuries, even death. We have become desensitized to this egregious injustice of mandated vaccination. People who dare question vaccine safety or claim that mandated vaccination is more about profiteering than our children's safety are often punished, threatened with having their children taken or

treated prejudicially for speaking up for their liberty or for acting to right what they know is wrong. WE THE PEOPLE are no longer allowed to think for themselves or self-govern our very own bodies and blood chemistry. The mass of pharmaceutical lobbyists has assured mandated vaccination continue in perpetuity for profit and that parents have no part in the vaccination decision; having no adequate ability to protect their children from perceived or actual vaccine induced harm. There is hope for WE THE PEOPLE and for our progeny and that is THE TWO STEPS OF CORRECTION. Much SAFER vaccines will be a direct result of the TWO STEPS!

All we need to do collectively, as individuals, one by one, is to stand up for our **SUPREME RIGHT OF SELF-PRESERVATION** through, informed consent/DENIAL; to deny a vaccination that is suspect or too controversial for injection. Demand to know all the chemicals used in the vaccine's production and act to protect your children from chemical insult. **Protect your children with the Self-preservation power to decide what healthcare is in your children's best health interest. Forbid the enforcing of harmful vaccines or vaccination that you deem not in your children's best interest or is too dangerous to inject.** Informed consent must steadfastly apply to vaccinations and vaccine producers must be held accountable and liable for vaccine induced injuries, made to compensate those proven injured by vaccination. Extreme caution is recommended to those contemplating a "suspect vaccination". **It is your life, it is your body to control and it is your own children that you must be FREE to protect!** The present state of chemically laced vaccines and the mandate that enforces **VACCINATION SLAVERY** is shameful and is really lawlessness. **TO ALLOW THE DECENCY AND NATURAL PROTECTION OF PARENTS' ENABLED TO REFUSE VACCINATIONS, WILL HAVE A PROFOUND POSITIVE IMPACT FOR SAFETY; IT WILL PROMPT SAFER VACCINES!**

Vaccine producers put all kinds of garbage in vaccines that treat the vaccine recipient like a toxic dump. They had to pushed and prodded into removing thiomersal (mercury) from vaccines and it is so abundantly, obvious that it should not, must not and need not be in vaccines; it is a commonly known neurotoxin. Neurotoxins trigger the faulty release of neurotransmitters causing a neurological hyperactivity. Attention deficit disorders and/or Autism have a main component of hyperactivity and/or inability to relax and be calm when one normally is meant to. When the body is supposed to be at rest either, voluntary or involuntary rest; it is interfered with because of the presence of chemical neurotoxins. Make no mistake, parents would NOT have heard, "DIAGNOSIS AUTISM" but for, the presence of abnormal to the body or unnatural to human biology unhealthy chemicalizations. Chemicals like Aluminum and other commonly found vaccine chemicals abnormalize the biochemistry and must NOT be in vaccines to have SAFER vaccines. Having less not more foreign to the body chemicals in vaccines is quintessential to developing a normal neurological and endocrine system. It is an essential to health understanding that vaccines must not be laced with toxins and/or foreign to the body chemicals. The TWO STEPS OF CORRECTION will push, prompt and force the makers of vaccines to produce vaccines with this essential to health understanding in mind! Chemicals for profit will no longer be in vaccines; making profits will not cloud judgement! The chains that hold children to suffer chemicalization will be broken by the TWO STEPS. Every strong hold on parenting will come down, every limitation will be released, and all the chains will be broken; allowing every fiber of parental protection to be reestablished. Children deserve the full dose of parental protection; they need ABUNDANT PARENTING!

Vaccination chemicals, artificial food additives such as, the food dyes, red dye 40, yellow dye 5 and 6 are just a few of the hurtful chemicals that are neurotoxins that cause synapse problems. Aspartame and other artificial sweeteners also contribute to the Autism spectrum causation. Preventing chemical exposures, which cause expecting mothers to become obese and/or stopping overweight people from continuing their circle of eating foods with harmful chemicals, are factors in Autism prevention. Realize that anything we put on our skin can be absorbed into the bloodstream, so please read the chemical contents and be the wiser for it. Parent's lathering up their babies at the beach with sun block may stop too much sun exposure but, please recognize **it is a chemical absorbable source.** Taking drugs in the sun is usually not wise however, do the proper amount of sun exposure without drugs can be very beneficial to staying healthy and recovering from health problems. **Conventional wisdom tells us to take major precaution and steps to avoid being consumed by all these chemicals that are deleterious neurologically.** Since, vaccinations are multiple and injected directly into babies, infants and children, it is of extreme importance and an emergency situation that we assure vaccines are produced without unnatural to the body, harmful chemicals. In order, to accomplish this health preservation and/or health assurances' **the TWO STEPS of CORRECTION must be taken.**

FDA chooses to be toothless; their position on all of these harmful chemicals is not to act to prevent us from exposure to any of these harmful chemicals but instead, merely conclude that all the children affected by these chemical exposures somehow, have a "unique sensitivity". The FDA blame our children for the Autism because they have "unique sensitivity" and not the reality that it is the chemicalization that is the main cause of the Autism epidemic. The prevention of the Autism epidemic could have been realized if only the FDA did not distract attention from the truth. **The truth is that all children have sensitivity to vaccine alien, unnatural to the body chemicals; it is a falsehood and distraction to state or attempt to put the blame on children and not the chemicalizations.** The FDA blinded the People from the major cause of Autism by pointing the belittling finger at the children and distracting the people from the truth that it is the chemicals. The contention that vaccine chemicals are not at all dangerous and/or harmful but rather, it is merely that there is some unique sensitivity that children have is a gross inaccuracy and an actual misleading. The term "unique" indicates that the FDA is confusing the public into thinking that only certain children are sensitive and that the blame is on the children and not the harmful chemicals. The truth that the chemicals of vaccines are the causative agent of Autism is brushed aside by calling children's weakness into the lime light of distraction.

The so called, "Vaccination Court" where it is very difficult to bring a case and get awarded damages from the "Master" (NOT A JUDGE AND NO JURY) continues to show just how injurious vaccine chemicalization is. Despite all its shortcomings and inequities of the

Vaccination Court, it has awarded mega-millions to vaccine induced injury victims. The proven injuries related to vaccination and the amount of money paid to those injured by vaccination clearly shows that vaccines do injure and at an alarming frequency and/or that the injuries are severe. In addition, there is a mounting mass of parents that have witnessed their children's health demise because of vaccinations that never take issue in the Vaccination Court. All of this has been suppressed; the toxic facts about vaccines has not been publicized as, it should. Despite the public not being properly or adequately informed about vaccines' toxic facts, many parents know that vaccines are not safe and want SAFER vaccines for their children.

Deep down in parent's bones is the need to protect their children; parents must be **FREE to refuse chemical infiltration** injections and/ or chemical exposure; this basic liberty will automatically trigger the need for vaccine producers to make SAFER vaccines. Parents must ensure their children's safety and that includes being enabled to refuse vaccination, chemical injections. The mandated vaccination law is in direct conflict with parental protection. **Perhaps, the FDA has forgotten the basic laws of chemistry or the rules of chemical engagement or reactions and outcomes and that the injection of unnatural body chemicals into tiny babies, little infants and small children is an inevitable poisoning of their blood and brain cells! It is vastly, important for parents to understand the negative to health propensities of unnatural to the body chemicals and protect their children accordingly! There is certainty that the abnormal to the human biology chemicals injected into children will react once injected and there is the uncertainty principle that can these abnormal reactions reach a level that will cause Autism or permanent abnormality. Parents by mal-law vaccination mandate must not be enforced to compromise children's chemistry.**

The truth is all our children have sensitivity to such, chemicals; it is the chemicals that injure that need to be brought into the spotlight of blame and causation. The FDA is too quick to blame children for their so called, "unique sensitivity" perhaps, it is the FDA's obvious bias toward the chemical industry or its close ties with Big Pharma is making the FDA's conclusion; the FDA conclusion is baffling at best. Children are not so inherently, different from each other to have drawn such, an erroneous conclusion. The FDA responses and their steadfast positioning and/or support for the vaccine industry or that the more chemicals the better positioning makes the FDA cohorts of the vaccination and chemical industry. One can conclude the FDA is colluding in a cover-up to stop vaccine chemicalization from being recognized as the true cause of Autism and is continually acting to protect the profiteering from vaccines. The FDA higher ups landing golden jobs at Big Pharma directly after their work at the FDA is a sign that we need to pay attention to!

The mandated vaccination law is not merely a regulatory support of the vaccine industry; it is an outright creation of guaranteed profiteering from an enslaved people that all must be subjected to suffer their children with vaccination; it is a medical monopoly! This pushed or mal Marshall law monopoly has resulted in UNSAFE vaccines where chemicals for profit, not safety are commonly found in vaccines! Drug Companies/Vaccine Producers and the FDA staff too often have a very close working relationship that can lead to bias or favors. There is a major conflict of interest because select workers for the FDA are offered very high paying jobs, working for the very Vaccine Producers/Drug Companies that they are supposed to police. One is COGNITIVELY CAPTURED to do what is in the best interest of vaccine producers or rather, not in the interest of the public when jobs/cash dangle in front of them; CONFLICT OF INTEREST and negative to safety spawns. The TWO STEPS will give parents back the control of children's welfare; REMEMBER, THEY ARE YOURS TO PROTECT! The mandated vaccination laws enfeeble parenting or parents right or ability to safeguard children, to protect offspring from abnormal to the body chemicalization.

Law must not deter, misdirect or nullify parents from refusing what parents deem too dangerous or too harmful vaccines from being injected into their children. Vaccine concoctions that have been proven to be laced with unnatural to human biology chemicals must not be enforced upon the people. To mandate vaccines that taint one's blood or manipulate one's blood chemistry with abnormal to human biology chemicals is a ruthless disregard of human life. Children's require the cautious guidance of their parents to best safeguard them from unwanted medical intervention or untrustworthy or corrupted by unnatural to human biology chemical vaccines; parental efficacious management best protects children! Parents protection of children's blood chemistry and/or health must not be negatively impacted by mal-law. The vaccination mandate enjoins parents to suffer children with vaccine chemicalizations that the parents object to and/or have determined are bad for the welfare of their children; it therefore, must be rendered illegal! By the fundamental maxims of true liberty, parents' obligations toward securing the well-being of their children must not be so, interfered with by for profit, mandated vaccinations. We must be forever vigilant not to subvert parents' power of protection of children. Parents need to be completely FREE to secure their children's life-giving natural chemistry. Law and the FDA must secure our liberty of parenting and allow children to benefit from it!

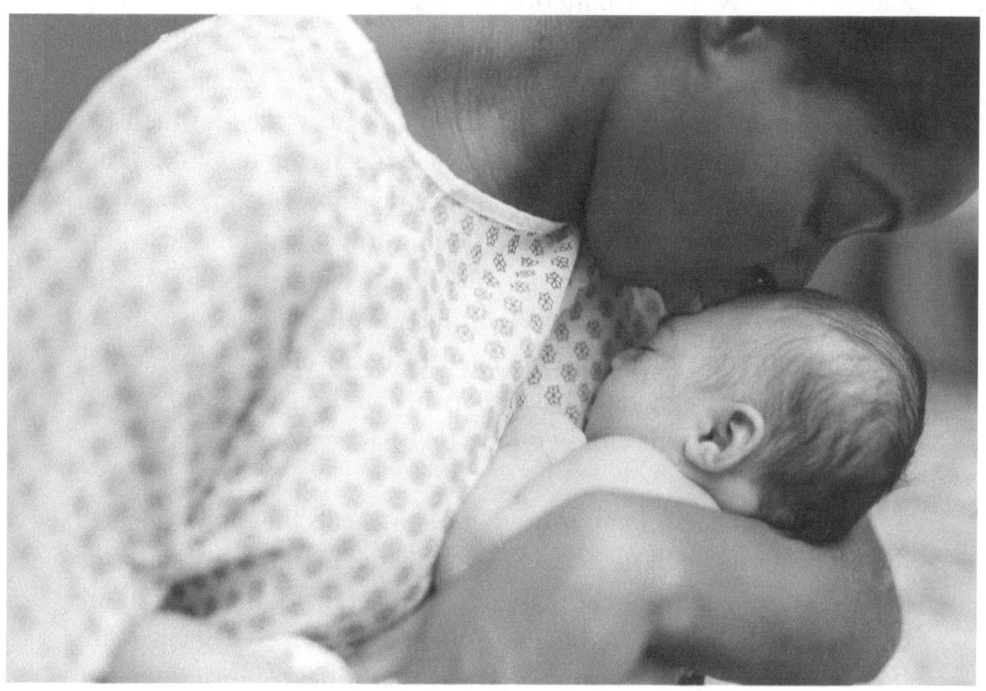

DO BE SURE YOU KNOW WHAT
CHEMICALS ARE IN VACCINES!

Instead of protecting our children from the transgressions of those who put unnatural to human biology chemicals that harm in vaccines, the FDA callously continues to display slated, one-sided judgments. FDA has a rigid and unbending support of vaccinations on unsound grounds. They are a monstrously deceptive; they do not serve to protect us when they allow unnatural chemicalizations of children. The FDA appears to have a violent prejudice to anything natural or that does not serve to perpetuate profit for the drug industry. Perhaps, knowing that FDA employees have obtained very lucrative jobs and titles or the hope for potential better jobs is influencing judgement to be so, positively biased toward vaccine manufacturers at our children's health expense. Big Pharma provide a whopping 60% of the FDA's drug/vaccine review costs and that means most of the FDA funding comes from those they are supposed to be investigating; this is a huge conflict of interest. The FDA often receives over 700 MILLION FROM Big Pharma per year; the FDA knows who is buttering both sides of its toast. The FDA's conflicts of interest have infiltrated into GMO being treated with unfair pro bias at the public's safety expense for example: Michael Taylor, started as an attorney for Monsanto, then quickly worked for the FDA just long enough to draft the FDA's policies decreeing that GMOs are "generally recognized as safe" and are exempt from labeling, and then went *back* to Monsanto. They are pulling this off in broad daylight however, we are all asleep or stupidly blindly trust in the FDA. The CDC is under the same conflicts of interest; Big Pharma is sure to influence all concerned. **Parents need to be in charge** of children's vaccination welfare; parents have no such, conflicts! The good news is that we can assure our children have **SAFER** vaccines for **parents to choose**.

The FDA beats a loud drum that always beats the same tune and there will always be those that reflexively march to the beat of the same deafening drum. **It cannot be denied that expectant mothers and young children are being exposed to more chemicals than ever before. This increased chemical exposure makes it that much more imperative that we assure our children are not exposed to vaccine chemicals which are not indigenous to the body. Injected chemicalization is the worst kind of chemical exposure because it enters the body** unabated and quickly circulates to breach the blood brain barrier and thereby, dopes the brain cells with its full chemical payload. Children's chemical tolerance can be challenged prior to vaccination and the FDA needs to take this into account. Human Rights forbid the enforcement of unwanted vaccine CHEMICALIZATIONS. Vaccines should always be works in progress to achieve the highest degree of safety; the TWO STEPS OF CORRECTION applied to vaccination will achieve SAFER vaccines and instill that vaccine producers constantly strive for safety, always being on the verge of excellence. There is no valid excuse for abnormalizing children with unnatural to the human biology chemicals in vaccines such as, but not limited to thimerosal or aluminum; the TWO STEPS will assure such, abnormal to the body chemicals or chemicals for strict profit are not used.

The FDA is WRONGFULLY, being used to stamp out competition for Big Pharma. There is attempting to make vitamins something that can only be prescribed. You no longer will be able to state the truth that vitamins and minerals can be a cure or aide or PREVENT disease because if you do; it automatically subjects it to be categorized as a drug and THAT IS CRAZY. The FDA is trying to regulate that if it claims to cure and/or help in recovering from an ailment or disease, it must be classified as a drug and thereby, can only be prescribed; the public will no longer have free access; vitamins and minerals will no longer be able to be sold in stores. This is utter nonsense, vitamins come from food, in fact, it must be considered food. Vitamins keep you healthy and/or help make you healthy and PREVENT YOU FROM FAULTERING TO THE POINT THAT YOU HAVE NO CHOICE BUT TO TAKE CHEMICAL DRUGS. Because vitamins negate the need or decrease the need to spend money on drugs it is being subjected to unfair attacks and unwarranted or unjustified regulation. Important to health; vitamins are naturally utilized by the body whereas; drugs are chemicals are unnatural to the body and all have adverse side-effects. The FDA's true mode of operation is to assure the drug industry's welfare and not ours! We need liberty to access to natural remedies and not be overburdened to obtain needed or wanted vitamins or be forced to needlessly spend time and money go to the doctor to attain them. It is drugs and vaccines that need more FDA oversight; just **look at the Big Pharma induced opioid and vaccine CHEMICALIZATION epidemics.**

When it comes to the cause of Autism; **it is CHEMICALS that need to be blamed and not our children! YES,** children all have sensitivity toward toxic chemicals, but children's susceptibility cannot be corrected and is not the causation of Autism or health problems rather, it is the chemicals. What can and needs to be corrected is to stop using alien to human physiology, abnormal to one's biochemistry and unnatural to human biology chemicals in our children's vaccines! **STOP EXPOSING OUR CHILDREN TO CHEMICALS that all children are sensitive to that cause abnormal reactions and abnormality. Children's chemical geometry must not be manipulated by mandated vaccine CHEMICALIZATIONS. PARENTS MUST BE FREE TO REJECT INJECTIONS THAT ARE UNWANTED OR DEEMED DANGEROUS; SECURING THEIR CHILDREN'S PERFECTED NATURAL BIOCHEMISTRY!**

Biologically we are not that different from one another; all children are susceptible to HARMFUL UNNATURAL TO HUMAN BIOLOGY CHEMICALS. The more natural we keep our children's blood or biochemistry the healthier they will be for it. The less unnatural to human biology chemicals that surge through the bloodstream or distort the natural biochemistry that healthier children will be for it; the SAFER our children will be! Although, our children's level of exposure to unnatural chemicals differs; it is a biological accurate fact, that unnatural to the body chemical exposure is negative to the health of all children and that Autism is chemically induced. The level and/or degree of chemical exposure causing the consequential level and/or degree of negative to health results can be the only question. For the FDA to have so quickly and readily concluded that children develop problems from their exposure to chemicals merely because they are "uniquely sensitive" is so off base that it is suspect. It appears to purposely misdirect a proper concern about vaccine chemicals causing Autism; there needs to be laser focus on **the chemicals that our**

children are unwisely, being exposed to. The prevention of chemical exposure of our children will majorly help prevent Autism.

If the FDA were to conclude that the presence of chemicals in the body has anything even remotely to do with Autism the axe would fall, the truth be told, and the revelation revealed of the etiology of Autism; their Drug company cohorts would be in trouble and jog opportunity would disappear. The chemicals from all the vaccines that are pumped by injection into children's delicate blood are the major cause of Autism and a gamut of other health problems. To have allowed children to have been exposed to the mercury derivative thimerosal, a known neurotoxin is scandalous and to continue to allow children to be injected with unnatural chemicals should be considered gross negligence, reckless endangerment of children and/or is toxic corruption. **The chemicals of vaccines do cause harm and are the main etiology of Autism! It is all too common after being vaccinated to have a fever and the fever can be very high; this in itself is an alarm ringing loud and clear that the vaccine is causing injury. A high fever by itself could be a contributing factor in DIAGNOSIS AUTISM however, a fever in conjunction with unnatural to human biology chemicals from vaccines surging around in the body or blood is too much for a tiny baby, little infant or small child to survive healthy with.**

It is that the FDA which has the problematic unique sensitivity to anything that might interfere with its too close relationship with vaccine companies. The FDA appears to be colluding with Big Pharma and seems to with grant vaccine producers an out of jail card and is deaf, dumb and blind to the fact, that vaccines have been found to have toxic chemicals or chemicals which are unnatural to human biology; we should all be very concerned about it. By the FDA stating that children who are "uniquely sensitive" are adversely affected at least gives the public a degree of warning although, not the proper degree. The FDA should have completed their thought by clearly, stating that these children become Autistic. This can be considered definitive proof that the **FDA KNOWS vaccination chemicals cause Autism.** The truth needs to be told that all children have sensitivity and can be caused Autism; **it primarily depends upon the level and frequency of chemical exposure (CHEMICALIZATION).** Just as one cannot be half pregnant, one is pregnant or not and so, it is true with chemicals; chemicals either do cause Autism or they do not; and clearly, **chemicals do cause Autism.** The twisted words of the FDA still confirm that unnatural to the body vaccine chemicals cause Autism; end of story. **Do not let them alter your children's internal chemistry unless, you truly think it is in your children's best interest however, do consider vaccinating with SAFER vaccines, generated by the TWO STEPS.**

The FDA has been so inattentive to allow a mercury compound and/or other unhealthy chemicals to be used in vaccines and have hindered the truth that vaccine chemicals are the major cause of Autism; it marks their **duplicity and bias. Turning the blind eye toward Big Pharma's purposeful use of unnatural to human biology chemicals in vaccines and FDA's cooperative agenda to limit Big Pharma competition by making natural remedies require a prescription or be categorized as a drug if a vitamin or natural remedy claims to cure anything places collusion at the feet of the FDA.** Vaccine producers use of mercury and other chemicals in vaccines destroys the trust we naively, placed in them. In 2001, a U.S. Food and Drug Administration (FDA) study revealed that a **6-month-old** receiving the recommended complement of childhood vaccinations was exposed to total levels of **vaccine-based mercury TWICE AS HIGH AS THE AMOUNT CONSIDERED SAFE by the E.P.A. (Environmental Protection Agency) for diet,** it sounds too crazy to be true but, it is true. Vaccine producers conceived and achieved the use of the known neurotoxin mercury in our children's vaccines and that is unforgivable and hopefully unforgettable. Deranged minds, that irresponsibly, place mercury and other harmful chemicals in vaccines, **must NOT be trusted** with our children's welfare. **Children need to be protected by parents and to do so, parents 'must be FREE to refuse perceived of as, too dangerous vaccination; the FDA will not protect them!**

Let me be clear, it should not be said that vaccines cause autism rather, **it is the unnatural to human biology chemicals in vaccines that are unhealthy and primary cause of the Autism epidemic. It is the reckless endangerment of children to inject such, chemicals and to mandate the masses of children to be vaccinated with such, vaccine chemicalizations is to mandate mass child abuse by chemicalization.**

I do not know of one vaccine producer who has lost their job for irresponsibly, putting mercury in our children's vaccines; in fact, they may have received raises for the profits procured. You see, mercury despite its obvious negative to health attributes allows the vaccines a longer shelf-life, allowing the vaccines to sit on doctor's shelves and not spoil and thereby, assures more stock piling and less vaccine returns do to spoilage and that equals greater profit however, it is all at our children's health expense. We must get all the chemicals out; mercury is merely just one of health's stumbling blocks and/or ill-health's building blocks. It is the unnatural to the body vaccine chemicals that build the foundation for Autism. Autism is not idiopathic; it is the result of negative to health chemical infiltration! In order, to stop the prevalence of hearing "DIAGNOSIS AUTISM", the TWO STEPS must be initiated. Parents have every reason to be concerned! Our invaluable Human Right to protect our children and supreme CONSTITUTION need reawakening; the TWO STEPS will do that and more! We do not want to destroy the vaccination compliance; we want to improve vaccine safety by achieving much SAFER vaccines and thereby, make vaccinating a RATIONAL CHOICE.

The charity at SAFER vaccines.org wants to open the eyes of parents to the importance of proper or healthy chemicalization and be properly warned about the dangers of improper or unhealthy chemicalization. It is of ultimate importance to health that health giving biochemical geometry is respected and that the laws of chemistry of t and within the body is not transgressed by vaccine injected unnatural to human biology chemicalization. Contemplate how the chemicals within your baby work to develop health or CHEMICALIZATION Autism, respect and understand how the laws of chemistry apply to either produce health or spawn Autism. Unclean vaccines act to destroy health; we must act to GET THE CHEMICALS OUT to give our children SAFER vaccines! Persevere in securing your children's vital chemistry free of unhealthy unnatural to human biology chemicals and you will not hear, "DIAGNOSIS AUTISM". Be FREE TO REJECT INJECTIONS of bad chemicals. A law is unjust and unworkable if it attempts to SEPARATE WHAT IS INSEPERABLE! The mandated vaccination law acts to separate children from inseparable parental guidance and protection when parents want to protect their children from what parents determine is a too dangerous to inject vaccine injection and are forbidden by mal-mandate to do so. When parents who determine a vaccine is not in their children's best interest and would refuse but for the mal-vaccination mandate acts to separate what is inseparable (the parents' protective decision not to vaccinate with what parents deem a vaccine that is not in their children's best interest). The erroneous mandate fails because in practice it is an impermissible FORFEITURE of parenting, an egregious violation of parental Rights that denies the parental and human trait to protect children from a possible or actual harm.

It would be an extraordinary claim that the injection of unnatural to human biology chemicals such as, but not limited to thimerosal (mercury derivative) and aluminum is harmless without extraordinary proof of it being harmless. The law of chemistry dictates that such, chemicals will take part in the reactions within the body and thereby, spawn abnormal to the body reactions causing **ABNORMALITY** and that is why it is unacceptable for many parents to jeopardize their children with such, vaccines. If you understand the consequences of altering the health or life-giving biochemistry you will want to consider only vaccinating with **SAFER** vaccines. No scholarly, doctor would inject unnatural to the body chemicals into tiny babies, small infants and very young children and have the ignorant state of mind to tell parents, in all good health conscious that it will not cause disharmony with health and/or that it could not possibly contribute to or cause the spawning of Autism. Chemicals are either health's building blocks or stumbling blocks; unnatural to human biology vaccine chemicals are stumbling blocks of health and/or the building blocks or causation of **CHEMICALIZATION AUTISM. Again, more evidence that they attempt to put the blame on children instead, of properly putting the blame squarely on vaccine chemicalization is when they infer that people who are pre-disposed to have a mitochondrial dysfunction can develop autistic conditions following vaccination.** The current President of Merck's Vaccines Division, Julie Gerberding inferred just that but by doing so, she with the same breath confirmed to CBS

News when she was Director of the US Centers for Disease Control that vaccines do cause Autism:

"Now, we all know that vaccines can occasionally cause fevers in kids. So, if a child was immunized, got a fever, had other complications from the vaccines. And if you're predisposed with the mitochondrial disorder, it can certainly set off some damage. Some of the symptoms can be symptoms that have **characteristics of autism.***"* WHAT QUACKS LIKE A DUCK IS A DUCK = WHAT IS CHARACTERISTIC OF AUTISM IS AUTISM! Chemicals dictate health or AUTISM! Harmful chemicals must not be in vaccines. The chemical test for **SAFER** vaccines is the **Sanity Test**, if there are unnatural to human biology chemicals in a vaccine it fails. Some think to have an "**idiot test**" for the doctor, if the vaccine is laced with toxic chemicals the vaccine fails the Sanity Test and the doctor would be an idiot to inject it. If the doctor is unaware of the toxic fact, of what chemicals are in vaccines he fails the idiot test. **The blame should fall heavily on the vaccine producer and doctor if there are unnatural to human biology chemicals in the vaccine and the child suffers a vaccine induced injury.**

The above quote is an inadvertent confirmation that vaccines cause Autism! However, the statement does attempt to misdirect the causation by stating that the Autistic victim must have a fever and be pre-disposed to whatever; the truth is that ALL CHILDREN ARE PRE-DISPOSED TO HAVE ABNORMAL REACTIONS AND HAVE ABNORMALITY FROM INJECTECTED VACCINES THAT CONTAIN UNNATURAL TO HUMAN BIOLOGY CHEMICALS. There is no myth that vaccines cause harm there is only the stark reality that vaccines do cause harm. We can render vaccines to be a much more intelligent choice by commanding SAFER vaccines through the TWO STEPS OF CORRECTION. Vaccinations being mandated and Big Pharma acting irresponsibly by negligently producing its vaccines with unnatural to human biology chemicals has made vaccination an irrational choice and given parents legitimate fear of vaccination!

When you investigate what chemicals have been found in vaccines or why they got there it becomes abundantly, clear that we should not let our children's health and/or health decisions be dominated by vaccine producers or **Big Pharma's puppet politicians.** For your information, the EPA recommends that women of **CHILDBEARING** age eat no more than six ounces of albacore per week. Canned (white) tuna has more mercury than canned (light) tuna and swordfish contains the highest level of mercury so, do not eat it. What is interesting here is that the recommendation is directed at potential pregnancies however, **the protection is really for the eventual newborns. If the EPA is concerned over mercury exposure for pregnant mother' or rather, newborns; vaccine producers should have the requisite insight and concern. Parents' must have extreme concern over the slightest degree of mercury in vaccines or any unnatural to the body chemical!** In fact, the vaccine-based mercury was "twice as high as the amount considered safe by the E.P.A." therefore; the concern should be off the scale and a stopping point for using mercury by vaccine producers. Public outrage and outcry was the main reason why most of the mercury was removed from most vaccines. **Parents' of Autistic children upon learning that their children were injected with such, chemicals in vaccines become extremely, upset and many rightfully become outraged. Parents should not put their children's health in profit based, callous, careless, unconcerned, self-serving and/or incompetent hands! Be safe not sorry; vaccinate with only SAFER vaccines!**

The harm from injected mercury is exponentially worse than the ingestion of it; there is no comparison. When we ingest mercury from tainted food it is much more slowly absorbed and there is a good chance that our digestive and elimination system will to a degree of efficiency and effectiveness eliminate the harmful chemical or minimize its absorption. The full dosage of ingested mercury will not enter the blood whereas, injected vaccines that contain mercury or other unnatural to human biology chemicals go directly **into the body or blood and circulates quickly, to one's fragile and all-important brain, doping the brain cells with the unabated full chemical payload; this poses a much greater danger to brain cells and brain function.** Vaccine chemicals enter the bloodstream all at once and suddenly with the velocity its injection, wreaking havoc with chemical homeostasis and/ or health. Even someone who is not an expert of science can easily recognize that this is a severe danger. These chemicals enter all at once and with nothing to slow the absorption or decrease the amount of chemicals that enter the blood. Parents are wanting this abnormal to the body chemicalization stopped; they no longer are willing to put their children's welfare into the hands of such, chemical folly. **Parental responsibility has been awakened as, parents are demanding informed consent/DENIAL.** Parents recognize that they need to adequately protect their children so, parents want to hold the vaccine industry liable for vaccine induced injuries and thereby, children can begin to be properly protected!

How many chemical injection exposures will it take to cause Autism? No one can be certain however, the more injections the more the likelihood of Autism and the more toxic the chemicals the less exposure is required to bring about the onset of Autism. By the age of 2 a toddler would have to submit to being injected with 28 doses of vaccines according to the schedule of vaccinations recommended by the Centers for Disease Control and Prevention; this is an unreasonable command since, vaccines place our children in double jeopardy, reacting to the antigens inherent in vaccines and being polluted by the toxic chemicals found in vaccines. Add up all the chemical exposures and its array of chemicals from the 28 vaccines that are all injected by the very young age of 2, which interact to cause chemical chaos within our children and **DIAGNOSIS AUTISM** becomes a plaque. Gardasil vaccine is yet another chemical insult that will be recommended to be injected and eventually attempted to make mandatory. **Parents should do everything in their power to assure vaccines do not expose their children to unwanted, anti-health chemicals; the TWO STEPS OF CORRECTION is that assurance. Demand not to be a VACCINATION SLAVE!**

WARNING: A new vibration and/or insight about prenatal ultrasound; a Yale study recently, revealed that prenatal ultrasound can cause brain damage in the developing fetus. During fetal development, neurons of the brain migrate to their correct positions. In a study of 335 mice, the researchers found that the ultrasound waves interfered with the normal migration of the neurons in fetuses. The amount of money being made from ultrasound is staggering; this Yale study is already being suppressed and innocent expecting parents will likely, not be given this potentially life and/or health saving information. It is obvious to me that the energy or magnetic field disturbance and/or the sound waves rippling into fetuses from frequent ultrasounds can cause health problems. As an Autism prevention it is wise not have abundant ultrasounds or limit it to when it is only absolutely warranted; newborns need to have all the neurons in their brain in perfect position for optimum brain function. Vaccine chemicalization of the babies that have had many unneeded disruptive to neuron ultrasounds is more of a sure recipe for Autism. Medical intervention of unnatural to the body chemicalization is the main causation of the Autism epidemic and ultrasounds' is yet, another medical intervention that is an Autism cause. AUTISM IS MAINLY AN IATROGENIC DISEASE (physician induced)!

Most parents find themselves in disbelief that they are so restricted by mandated vaccination regulation that they cannot decide what is best for their own flesh and blood or protect their children from what parents might deem too dangerous to inject vaccines. Parents are becoming logic stricken; they can add 1 and 1 and know that it is unwise in fact, outright wrong and dangerous to the health of their children to inject unnatural to human biology chemicals. People want the benefit of vaccines without being chemically compromised if they undergo vaccination! With all these chemicals in vaccines our children face the danger of a critical mass chemical overload and syndrome with each injection. Autism could be a vaccination away! We must be ever so careful not to alter the normal chemistry of the bloodstream, brain and body and/or tip the chemical scale to its tipping point, the point of creating a critical chemical mass syndrome. Over time the multiple vaccinations can interact spawning abnormal bio mutations. If foreign to the body chemicals continue to be pumped into children's blood the Autism epidemic will not decrease. Stop putting mercury in childhood vaccines was a step in the right direction however, we must not stop there; we must **CLEAN-UP VACCINES** to achieve **SAFER** vaccines. Steer clear of chemical infiltration particularly; injected chemicals and you will protect your children from neurological disturbances and prevent hearing "DIAGNOSIS AUTISM". Be vigilant to protect your child's natural geometric chemistry and they will naturally be healthy; the possibility of Autism becomes highly remote!

Anyone, with basic knowledge of chemistry can understand the danger of injecting unnatural to human biology chemicals. Most, if not all, people who understand the laws of chemistry agree or are on the same page, that to inject such, chemicals are hazardous to health. There is even controversy among the experts as to whether it is in children's best health interest to expose them to all the varying **vaccine antigens especially, when toddler's immune systems are just starting to come on line. Exposure to vaccine's antigens could severely strain an immature immune system and cause the immune system to malfunction perhaps, permanently.** This is analogous to a very young person who foolishly, lifts too much weight in a poorly supervised or unsupervised workout; the under-developed youth could easily become strained, injured or herniated. Just as it is unwise to workout with heavy weight when very young or rather, wiser to slowly build up your ability to lift heavy weights; one could injure the immune system by forcing it to work out or work to concur the antigens of vaccines. One can strain an immature developing immune system with vaccine injected antigens. This onslaught of antigens when combined with the presence of unnatural vaccine chemicalization is much more harmful or problematic. **Parents need to be FREE to weigh-out the pros and cons of vaccinations and must not be enforced to vaccinate! When parents detect a danger to injecting the chemicals of vaccines and/or have determined that vaccination is not in their children's best interest; no vaccination should be given or legally can be allowed to be given. Those children that have Autism are chemically compromised and parents must be FREE to stop further VACCINE CHEMICALIZATION; this prevention gives the best chance at recovery!**

Life without boundaries is chaos and parents not placing boundaries on what their children can or shall be injected with leads to their children's welfare chaos and/or Autism. Why vaccines manufacturers risk children's welfare or place their health in chaos by putting unnatural to the biology chemicals in vaccines is troubling and raises many questions. When it comes to vaccine contents or its lack of safety there are towering questions-questions too tall for us to see past, even when we stand on tiptoe. Rather, be safe than sorry; do consider vaccinating however, only vaccinate with **SAFER** vaccines! **How many chemical injections can your children withstand? Does 28 doses of vaccines by age 2 concern you? What number of enforced vaccine doses of chemicals is cause for concern to the rational parent is it, 1, 2, 28, 38, 50, 100 or more? How many chemicals would you let your children be exposed to before you COMMAND "STOP" AND TAKE PROTECTIVE ACTION? CHEMICALIZATION** Autism can be one injection away! The least toxic chemicals your children are exposed to the lower the chances of hearing, DIAGNOSIS AUTISM. The enforcement of even one injection is outrageous and must be forbidden. Live FREE to reject injections. Protect your children from unwanted chemical exposure; protect them from Autism, as you see fit. One enforced chemicalization is one to many, in the eyes and hearts OF THE FREE. Overzealous vaccination advocates appear to think that if they gave so many vaccines that it replaced one's blood completely that it would be fine and would cause no health problems. Make no mistake, health is dependent upon proper chemicalization (the building blocks of health) and the prevention of unnatural to human biology chemicalization (stumbling blocks)!

Further, excellent reason to demand your fundamental healthcare **Right to refuse an unwanted vaccine chemicalization is that many doctors themselves refuse to have it.** Doctors are supposedly more in the know, they realize that the benefit of the vaccination are vastly, outweighed by the fact, that vaccines come with multiple **risks from the bad CHEMICALS INHERENT.** In the February 1981 Journal of the American Association found that **66 percent of pediatricians REFUSED to take the rubella vaccine and an astounding 90 percent of obstetricians REFUSED.** Moreover, during interviews with many doctors, who prefer to remain anonymous for fear of being ostracized, they revealed that they have not had their own children vaccinated or completely vaccinated **because of the possibility of harm and doctors confessed they falsified immunization records to make their children appear to be vaccinated.** In the British Medical Journal, January 27, 1990, a survey of 598 doctors revealed **over 50 percent of** the doctors REFUSED hepatitis vaccine, despite that they belonged to the high-risk group and were strongly urged to undergo vaccination. It is unjust and inequitable for children to be enforced into vaccine chemicalization especially, when the parents want to refuse it! If doctors were presented with SAFER vaccines, they would less likely refuse. The TWO STEPS of CORRECTION will increase safety and cause less fear of vaccination.

The medical profession itself apparently, thinks vaccinations should not be enforced upon children by a government vaccination mandate. On November 2nd, 2000 at their 57th annual meeting in St. Louis, Missouri, members of the Association of American Physicians and Surgeons (AAPS), unanimously passed a resolution, without a single vote against the resolution, calling for, "a moratorium on vaccine mandates and for physicians to insist upon truly informed consent for the use of vaccines." However, even though doctors unanimously do not want vaccinations given without the true consent of parents and that vaccine quality suffers because of the mandate; the big business and deep pockets of Big Pharma commands that children callously continue to be handcuffed to be vaccinated by vaccination mandate. For profit, vaccine manufacturers' want to keep us or rather, our children ENSLAVED to be vaccinated and pave the way for more and more vaccines for profit to be mandated. They want to keep children ENSLAVED to be vaccinated to assure mega profiteering from vaccine sales produced by enforced vaccinations. They want to assure vaccines sales continue to grow undisturbed and uninterrupted. It does not want its profit-making machine to be messed-up by free thinking parents that act to protect children from unwanted vaccine CHEMICAL harm.

The AAPS Executive Director Jane Orient, MD had two statements that are important, the first is "Our children face the possibility of death or serious long-term adverse effects from mandated vaccines that aren't necessary or have very limited benefits." The second is "AAPS believes that parents, with the advice of their doctors, should make decisions about their medical care-not government bureaucrats. This resolution affirms that position." Wow, these ethical doctors put patients' Rights above profiteering; we should salute them! PARENTS' NEED TO RECOGNIZE what these ethical doctors' recognize! Mandated vaccination is at odds with the Parental Right to decide what is best for their children, to protect their children from unwanted or perceived of as too dangerous to inject vaccine chemicalizations and with the entire medical association unanimous voted moratorium on vaccine mandates and for physicians to insist upon truly informed consent for the use of vaccines. If mandated vaccination were not so unconscionably profitable, it would not be mandated; money is overpowering liberty and our safety. If people cannot refuse vaccination there will be a dominate and controlling mechanism to put CHEMICALS FOR PROFIT in vaccines that are not safe for injection; we must be FREE TO REJECT INJECTIONS! Protect your children's vital life-giving biochemistry!

The chemicals within us dictate our level of health.

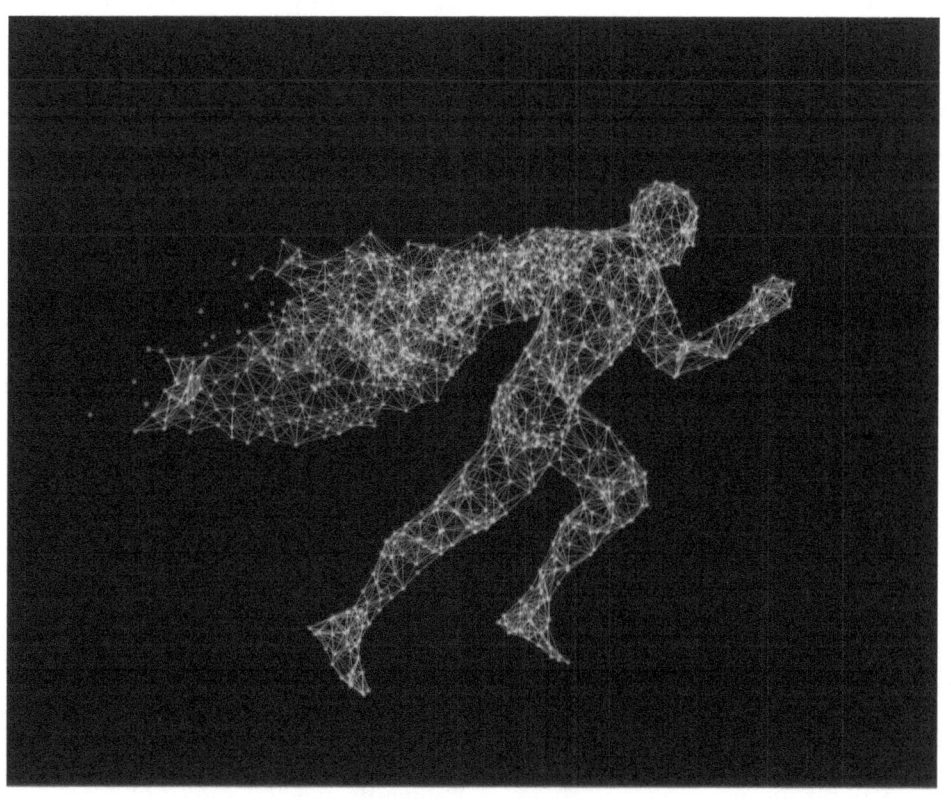

Super health requires a normal biochemistry.
Inject only SAFER vaccines.

People' need to stand up for the Right to protect their children from unwanted chemical injection exposures and assure vaccine quality through informed consent or rather, informed DENIAL; to bring vaccines under reasonable restraints and safety. Let us bring about an equitable and just vaccination delivery system based upon safety first; brought on and secured by PARENTAL DECISION AUTHORITY and SAFETY SATISFACTION COMPULSION! The real reason vaccinations are mandated is not for our children's best interest but rather, for corporate interest. ASSuring vaccine sales with a definite endless market of children's arms to stick millions of vaccination needles into and inject its vaccines means endless mega-profiteering. They want parents to have no Right to refuse any of its chemical vaccine injections so, it can profit without interference or restriction. Corporate lobbyists have infiltrated our legal system, bastardized the legal process by manipulating law-making to serve corporate self-interest and not our children's best interest. IF THERE WERE NO PROFIT TO BE MADE BY MANDATING VACCINATIONS; THERE WOULD BE NO MANDATES! It is in the best interest of children to preserve their natural chemical geometry; corporate greed is at odds with this interest!

WARNING: yet another vaccine mandate is well underway or rather, sick mindedly underway, … in the month of October 2011, the Advisory Committee on Immunizations Practices, that advises the U.S. Centers for Disease Control and Prevention, voted to recommend ROUTINE use of Gardasil in 11 to 12 – year – old BOYS. Previously, the Gardasil vaccine was only recommended for girls; now they are additionally, attempting to profit from injecting boys as well as girls. Parents should think twice before having girls injected and think more than that about having their boys vaccinated with a Gardasil chemical concoction. No one should be mandated to be vaccinated! Injecting boys with more chemical toxins and/or Gardasil vaccine venom is a giant step in the wrong direction. Exposing children to more chemicals while their young bodies are growing and maturing and/or going through rapid cell differentiation and metabolic changes is further recipe for Autism. Children's optimum health is dependent upon the proper natural chemistry; to further manipulate or distort it with more vaccines is too dangerous. Gardasil has unnatural to human biology chemicals in it and is therefore, too dangerous. To end the slippery slope of more and more vaccinations and the epidemic of DIAGNOSIS AUTISM; the TWO STEPS OF CORRECTION need to be implemented!

The Gardasil vaccination is part of the ongoing **slippery slope of vaccinations** as, there is further attempt to turn our children into **vaccine pin cushions**. It wrongfully assumes our children will need vaccine protection due to mere conjecture of sexual promiscuity. It presumes an increased risk of human papilloma virus from having sex with multiple partners. It totally discounts parental moral teachings and egregiously removes parents from the all-important decision over whether their children will need Gardasil's supposed protection. Parents talking to their children about the birds and the bees or safe sex becomes a moot point. According to Gardasil advocates children will all grow to have sex before marriage and/or have sex with multiple partners. Parental responsibility, authority and/or their Right to raise children and protect children according to one's private and personal beliefs and knowledge is under attack. There is alien, unnatural to the body chemicals in the Gardasil vaccine that parents need to access in deciding what is best for their children. **Recommending even more vaccine chemicalizations than the already commanded childhood vaccine chemicalizations is further placing your children in harm's way. Chemically induced health problems and/or CHEMICALIZATION AUTISM can be an injection away! To make Gardasil mandated is to take the health disaster created from mandated vaccinations and turn it into more of a catastrophe!**

How much vaccine chemical exposure does your child have to be enforced to endure until you say "STOP"? Under what set of circumstances would you demand parental decision authority and satisfaction? Is there a chemical content point that would make you prevent the vaccine chemicalization and demand safety and/or SAFER vaccines for your children? In order, to STOP THE CHEMICALIZATION MADNESS parents must instill the needed CORRECTIVE TWO STEPS. Act to prevent AUTISM; do not be ENSLAVED to compromise your children's chemical integrity!

Be on the alert for any attempted violation of your parental Rights or devaluation of the parent/child relationship. Your vested natural parental responsibilities include protecting your children from chemicalization poisons or yet another egregious mandated vaccine. There is plan that Gardasil can be given not only **without parental informed consent permission but also, WITHOUT PARENTAL KNOWLEDGE.** The Gardasil vaccine will test the publics complacency in allowing their children to be further entrenched into **vaccination SLAVERY** and will take it a giant step further in the wrong direction in that the vaccine is being proposed to be delivered **WITHOUT PARENTAL KNOWLEDGE.** Parents, not government, should decide if any vaccine can be delivered! There must be parental permission to vaccinate. Vaccinations must not be enforced upon us; IT IS AN ABUSE OF GOVERNMENTAL POWER THAT MUST END!

Vaccination of children must only be given if the parents are convinced that the vaccination is in the best interest of their children. No harmful chemicals in vaccines means the healthier children will be! Children are much better off not being exposed to unnatural to the body chemicals. Parents must remain on guard, turned on, tuned in and tapped in, being constantly vigilant to assure their children's safety. To best assure children's safety the vaccination decision must be in the caring good hands of parents. **Government has failed to get vaccines right or are safe and yet, it still mandates vaccinations. Mandated vaccination is more for the benefit of Big Pharma than it is in the best interest of children. Parents need to be enabled to refuse unwanted vaccination, to best protect their children as, this enablement will get vaccines right; making sure vaccines are SAFE. We must be FREE not to be violated with unwanted medical intervention especially if it disrupts or distorts or alters the natural chemical geometry of the body or biochemistry. Vaccines that are not SAFER vaccines have a strong tendency to abnormalize the much-needed natural biochemistry. A blood chemical contamination results from vaccine chemicalization that infiltrate the body and blood with unnatural to human biology chemicals.**

In addition, to the risk of chemical exposure from vaccines, there is major concern that vaccinations are a one size fits all approach.

It is the author's strongest opinion that dosage requirements should be determined on an individual basis. It is unwise that gender, age, weight differential or state of health does not factor into vaccine dosage or timing of delivery. Medicine is at its best when it is specific to the patient or the patient's needs and it is at its worst when it does not. Mass vaccination based upon mass general dosages is medicine at its worst; vaccination needs to be individualized to prevent injury. Mandated vaccination is not only the practice of BAD medicine; it is the government practicing medicine without a license. It also, perpetuates less need for quality control and thereby, has produced unsafe vaccines. SAFER vaccines charity takes the darkness of not knowing what negative to health contents are in vaccines or not knowing its ill-health consequences and floods light on it; giving insight on what harmful unnatural to human biology chemicals are in vaccines and how to obtain SAFER vaccines for the safety and well-being of children.

Producers of vaccines do not have the requisite compassion nor motivation to protect our children from chemicalization harm; they care not, do not listen to parental concerns about vaccine's being too dangerous due to unnatural to human biology chemical content. The fact, that vaccines continue to have unnatural to human biology chemicals despite injuries that are vaccine induced and parents' rational concerns and its total disregard for the basic laws of chemistry or how its abnormal to the body chemicals cause abnormality; it is more than evident that Big Pharma, its masses of lobbyists and its puppet government officials have not, and will not, protect children properly. Implement the TWO STEPS OF CORRECTION and it will assure SAFER vaccines and arrest parental fear! One thing is certain that parents need to do to safeguard their children and that carefully consider what it is that you are contemplating injecting into their vital blood and body. However, many times even when you think the contents are safe; it turns out it is harmful. The golden rule or the "SANITY TEST for vaccines is, if it has unnatural to human biology chemicals it must be considered unhealthy, too dangerous to risk injection and is likely to injure!

You never know what you are unleashing from a **MASS** vaccination

CHEMICALIZATION program. In a May 11, 1987, London Times article entitled, 'Smallpox vaccine triggered Aids virus' The World Health Organization is studying scientific evidence that immunization with smallpox vaccine Vaccinia awakened the dormant human immune defense virus infection (HIV). Throughout the world, the greatest spread of HIV infection coincides with the most intense immunization programs. The **MASS** chemicalizations from the **MASS** vaccinations **are ruled by the LAWS OF CHEMISTRY thus, MASS reactions and abnormal formations unnatural to the body result**. There is also, mounting evidence that vaccines do not protect children as they are drummed up to. It is terrible that vaccines are enforced upon us and this is cause enough to make vaccination strictly voluntary however, the growing evidence that vaccinations do not adequately protect what they are supposed to protect; make the enforcement of vaccinations even more outrageous. In the November 21, 1990, (JAMA), Journal of the American Association had an article that stated, "Although, more than **95 percent** of school-aged children in the US are vaccinated against measles, large measles outbreaks continue to occur in schools and **MOST CASES in this setting occur among previously vaccinated children**." The efficiency and effectiveness of vaccines is called into question; the public needs to be made aware of this. Perhaps, if they GET THE CHEMICALS OUT, making SAFER vaccines, the vaccine would work better. Those **not exposed** to vaccine chemicals are obviously, **more resilient; healthier**. Freedom of choice and fundamental liberty of deciding what is best for one's children requires that parents be **FREE** to make an educated decision on a vaccine and **BE FREE TO REJECT INJECTION.** If parents deem the vaccine not in their children's best interest or too dangerous to inject the parents decision must be respected and the vaccine not given!

The Community Disease Centre, UK, reported that in the UK between 1970 and 1990, over 200,000 cases of whooping cough occurred in **fully vaccinated children**. In the July issue of the New England Journal of Medicine a study revealed that over **80 percent of children** less than five years of age who had **contracted whooping cough had been FULLY vaccinated**. According to, The Lancet, September 21, 1991, in Oman between 1988 and 1989, a polio outbreak occurred amongst thousands of **FULLY** vaccinated children. **The region with the LOWEST attack rate had the LOWEST vaccine coverage.** Parents' make the vaccination decision; **DO NOT BE enforced and/or ENSLAVED to vaccinate your children.** The validity or effectiveness of vaccines is important to the vaccination decision. The **less** unnatural to human biology chemicals equals the more efficient and effective the biochemistry. It is logical that children who have been chemically compromised by unsafe vaccines are rendered more susceptible to childhood disease because of it. Chemicals within effect health resiliency!

When my auto mechanic asked me why his fully vaccinated infant son got the measles and had all kinds of health problems I explained to him that if the vaccine was not a **SAFER** vaccine that it had all kinds of unnatural to human biology chemicals in it that mixed with the once pure and natural homogeneous biochemistry and that it caused abnormal reactions; causing abnormality and that one is less resilient to childhood disease because of it. My mechanic understood what I said and compared it to what happens to a car when its brake line fluids or its steering power fluid becomes contaminated; it fails because the brake fluid or the steering power fluid is contaminated with chemicals that are not brake or powering steering fluid chemicals that are part of the chemistry needed to brake or assist steering. The brakes and the powering steering can fail because the chemical makeup of the fluid is altered or abnormalized. This demonstrates a good understanding of the situation; that the law of chemistry applies to function, metabolism and/or if one is to be healthy or is being rendered sick or Autistic! I went to eat at a world-renowned restaurant and when the great chef's creation was served I was overwhelmingly pleased. I spoke to the chef about health and how foreign to the body chemicals in vaccines cause Autism. The chef showed me that he had a clear understanding of what I was saying when he responded with the following, "when I am recreating a meal it requires a set range of ingredients to have the same great taste and palate consistency that my patrons expect and appreciate; if a single ingredient is off or a foreign to the recipe ingredient is mistakenly added the outcome can be disastrous, the meal is not the same, it is unacceptable, ruined." The key to outcome is the chemicals that dictate it; unnatural to the body chemicalization "ruins" health.

There is also evidence of cases of "non-polio paralysis" from over-dosing children, too much polio vaccination or intense immunization practices. In addition, CBS News, February 24, 2014, by Ryan Jaslow, 20 – 25 children became paralyzed and had injury to their spinal columns; **eerily similar to polio and with polio like symptoms**. The polio vaccination likely, caused the so called, "non-polio paralysis; **it is polio, with a new misleading name**. Prior to the advent of the polio vaccination; **these vastly similar signs and symptoms would be diagnosed, POLIO**. We know chemicals cause cancer; we need to also, recognize that chemicals cause **AUTISM!** It is not too long or high of a bridge to cross to conclude the danger of injecting unhealthy chemicals. Your children need and deserve the needed for health chemicals and the best vaccines possible. With liberty of vaccination decision, we can steer clear of unwanted chemicalization; and protect our children from chemicalization harm.

If one is not free to decide to do what he or she will with one's body or parents cannot refuse a needling skin piercing and injection of vaccine chemicalization then we are suffered with VACCINATION SLAVERY! This slavery violates our Right to be left alone and annihilates one's liberty to Self-determine healthcare and has caused vaccines to become dangerous chemicalizations. ABOLISH VACCINATION SLAVERY and it prompts clean vaccines; GET THE CHEMICALS OUT! The universal laws of chemistry apply to all the vaccine chemicals so, let us act to get the unnatural to the body chemicals out. **Alien/foreign to the body chemicals of vaccines are contaminants to the bloodstream.** The fact that vaccines are injected directly into our children's sensitive body and blood and the exposure is all at once is reason for extreme caution and is excellent reason for the condemnation of vaccines that contain unnatural to human biology chemicals. Liberty to refuse promotes **SAFER** vaccines!

To prevent parents from ever hearing, **"DIAGNOSIS AUTISM"**, parents must be enabled to weigh-out the risks of not vaccinating as, compared to the inherent risks of vaccinating. If parents are not convinced of the safety of a vaccine or if they determine there is too great a risk of health degeneration or Autism, then parents must be **FREE** to protect their children by refusing the vaccination. There must be no legal pressure or any coercion to deter parents from protecting their children. In addition, if a child is diagnosed with Autism, Parents must be **FREE** to seek legal action against the Vaccine Producers when parents accuse it of negligent production of a vaccine that may have caused their child's chemistry to be compromised to any degree and/or caused their child harm and/or Autism. The Autism epidemic is mainly caused by the injection of unnatural to human biology chemicals found in vaccines; the primary prevention of CHEMICALIZATION AUTISM is the preservation of one's natural and normal biochemistry. For the welfare of children; Be FREE to REJECT INJECTIONS!

When you are vaccinated with a vaccine that is laced with unnatural to human biology chemicals you definitely, are faced with the unhealthy chemical distortion or abnormality caused by it whereas, if one is not vaccinated there is good probability that they either will not get childhood disease or that if they do get childhood disease they will completely recover from it or may actually become immunologically stronger for it and at the same time have a lifetime immunity because of it. The best scenario is to have SAFER vaccines to choose when weighing out the pros and cons of vaccinating verses not vaccinating. Facing the very real risks of vaccine chemical exposure verses the conjectural, theoretical or remote risk of incurring childhood disease must be decided by parents; not government. Government should not be making our health decisions. The elements required for optimum health and the factors that destroy health should be considered. Nutrition, chiropractic and other natural healthcare help enable the body to fight off disease or aid in recovery and super antibiotics help prevent childhood disease from being so destructive. There must be freedom to discern the options available and the risks inherent. Mandated vaccination is now antiquated law, unworkable law and has caused vaccines quality to fall to the wayside and/or harbor chemicals for profit, not safety. Law must not enforce chemical injection especially, if parents determine it not in children's best interest.

Parents want their liberty **TO DECIDE**; to weigh out the remote possibility of a childhood disease injuring their child verses the known and unknown injuries from vaccine chemicalization exposure. The logical negative health consequences of exposing children to the vaccine chemicals and antigens of 28 doses by the age of 2; must be allowed to be taken into **SERIOUS** consideration. **Parents should have the Right to protect their children from contamination and/or deny unwanted suspect vaccinations. The contamination is pertinent to health issues and the infraction of our Rights is pertinent and controlling to the legal issues! Parents need to do what they think is right by their children, do what it is they think is in their children's best interest and refuse anything that might cause "DIAGNOSIS AUTISM".** One can only imagine the negative to life affects of being enforced to inject your children with a vaccine that is considered unsafe however, one cannot imagine the anguish, the devastation perpetrated upon parents that are coerced or enforced to submit their children for unwanted vaccine chemicalization when their children suffer vaccine induced injury. Children's lives are at stake; we must do what is needed to assure SAFER vaccines!

Before you acquiesce with infiltrating your children with unnatural to the body vaccine chemicalizations realize that not only will the presence of these chemicals disrupt the normal reactions and bio-production of the body but also, the chemical environment in and around your cells can set the agenda for your genes and/or cellular function. **Genetic perversion, abnormal function, health degeneration and Autism can result.** The chemicals of vaccines can alter genes' behavior. It is far better to safeguard our children's internal environment by not exposing them to chemically laced vaccines. Vaccine Producers must be prompted to not use anti-health chemicals. We must not inject unnatural to the body chemicals. We must be **FREE** to prevent it. **FREEDOM** to pursue optimum health by pursuing optimum chemistry requires the **LIBERTY to deny unwanted chemicalization!** The plague of **DIAGNOSIS AUTISM** is fueled by injections of unnatural to human biology chemicalizations.

Children are becoming disconnected with nature. Children are induced to think that it is perfectly, natural to take pills or be injected with multiple vaccines and to be totally dependent upon medical intervention. Parents must work hard at protecting their children from the constant media blitz to take drugs for everything. Never have children been prescribed so many medicines and take so many illicit drugs; unchecked prescribed drug taking has increased illicit drug taking. **The key to preventing Autism is to prevent chemical exposure especially, injected chemicalizations. The key to Autism recovery is to stop further chemical exposure, rid the body of toxic chemicals and assure the proper levels of vitamins and minerals that are health's building blocks. Not injecting anti-health chemicals prevents Autism. Live FREE to follow your own healthcare agenda and/or live a natural life.** To curtail the Autism epidemic and prevent hearing, "DIAGNOSIS AUTISM" we must ABOLISH VACCINATION SLAVERY by instilling the TWO STEPS OF CORRECTION.

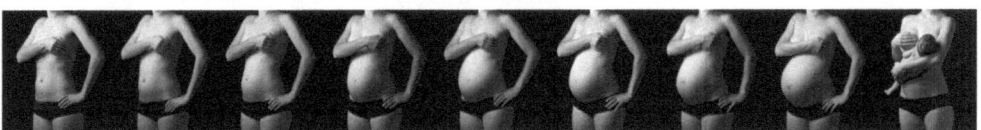

As your pregnancy progresses make sure you are not internalizing unnatural to human biology and abnormal to human development chemicals.

It is obvious that what we eat has major health consequences and **WHAT WE INJECT HAS EVEN MORE HEALTH CONSEQUENCES!** You would not allow your children to eat some of the chemicals found in vaccines so, why allow your children to be violated by injection with the harmful chemicals that have been found in vaccines? Know what chemicals are in the vaccine being pointed at your children for injection and act to protect your children from what is a **CHEMICALIZATION HARM**. Vaccination was made for man, not man for vaccination. Vaccination were created and established as a benefit for people. The advocates of Big Pharma, however, have turned this good gift into a weighty obligation under vaccination mandate. Parents have the sovereign authority to determine how vaccination delivery should be practiced; there must not be mandates that command parents to submit their children to suffer unwanted vaccine chemicalizations or even command wanted vaccinations. I tell you, if you allow your children to be chemically compromised that it will alter their vital biochemistry and thereby, cause abnormal reactions and/or abnormality. A critical mass chemicalization syndrome can spawn **CHEMICALIZATION AUTISM**. There are too many stumbling blocks of health in vaccines that are not **SAFER** vaccines. Perhaps the greatest positive health measures are to assure your children are receiving their needed for optimum health level of vitamins, mineral and pure water (the building blocks of health) and to avoid bad chemicalization especially, the injection of vaccines that carry unnatural to human biology chemicals (the stumbling blocks of health).

Understanding how the body works and the consequences of injecting into the body vaccines' unnatural to human biology chemicals, illuminates the cause of the Autism epidemic. The atom is the smallest particle (smallest unit of matter) that takes part in a reaction. Atoms combine to form compounds. Chemical compounds can generally be classified into two broad groups: molecular compounds and ionic compounds. Molecular compounds involve atoms joined by covalent bonds and can be represented by a variety of formulas. Ionic compounds are composed of ions joined by ionic bonding. What keeps the atoms together is bonding which is when atoms share electrons. A law of chemistry says that chemical reaction rearranges atoms into a new product. Chemical bonds are made or broken in order to create a new molecule. The presence of unnatural to human biology chemicals in the body can spawn alien to the body products that are not indigenous to human metabolism or physiology or biology. Chemicals change temperature and pH levels, affecting amino acid or enzyme activity or function. It is unwise to have chemicals in vaccines that are not within the biochemistry of the human and it is more unwise for noncarbon chemicals or noncarbon chemical compounds to be in vaccines. **If you distort the chemical biosphere of your baby, infant or child expect abnormality! The unnatural injected chemicals will become part of children's cells, enzymes and/or proteins.**

Vital bioproduction's of the body and their proper functioning require the proper geometric chemistry! **The biochemistry within our** cells and the environmental biochemistry surrounding cells is crucial to health and/or the prevention of CHEMICALIZATION AUTISM. The normal biochemistry or original reactants and final products of the chemically dependent bioreactions can be altered by introducing **unnatural to human biology chemicals.** Chemistry's collision theory is that increased motion of chemicals means more collisions in a system and that means more combinations of molecules from bouncing into each other. Because vaccines are injected rapidly into a rapidly flowing circulatory system, the moving unnatural to human biology vaccine chemicals spawn more abnormality as it collides in the circulatory system. If you have unnatural to human biology vaccine chemicals colliding with each other and with the normal to human biology chemicals intrinsic to the body there will be more possible combinations than what is normal; consequently, there is a higher chance that the molecules will complete abnormal to the body reactions, creating renegade or abnormal to human biology production and interference with normal production. The reaction will happen faster which means the rate of these abnormal to the body reactions will increase. Homeostasis is reliant upon maintaining the normal environment of the cells and that includes the chemicals inside and that surround the cells. Metabolism is the total of all the chemical reaction you need to survive and/or be optimally healthy. Abnormalize reactions and abnormalize production and thereby, it spawns abnormality and/or Autism. Be a body detective and seek all sources of unnatural to the body chemicalization to eliminate its exposure to children **especially, injected infiltrations of chemical compounds.**

The slightest change to your biochemistry can have major impact on health. Just look at what happens when you take prescription drugs; the chemicals have major impact. For example, when you take a steroid chemical formulation it is slowly destroying your internal organs; when you get older, you can have kidney and liver problems and you can even die from overuse. Literally, every chemical drug formulation has adverse side-effects and/or causes health problems. It is understood that unnatural to the human biology chemicals can cause cancer. Be warned: the same type of chemicals which can cause cancer can cause Autism. Injecting unnatural to human biology chemicals from vaccines is the leading cause of Autism. We must be **FREE** to prevent our children from being abnormally chemicalized; we need **SAFER** vaccines. Never take drugs to enhance your body. Those athletes are hurting their bodies. They can't see it, because it is slowly destroying their internal organs and not the muscles. Never vaccinate with a vaccine that has unnatural to human biology chemicals; you may not see its negative to health impact immediately, but its negative to health impact is there. **Parents rapped in their parental supreme authority and/or constitutional prerogatives have control over whether a vaccine will or will not be injected;** trumping any mandated vaccination law or for mere profit regulation! We must not expose children to unnatural to the body chemicals such as, but not limited to, heavy metals because **it is a poison to enzymatic activity. Heavy metal ions react with S-H group of cysteine bonds, forming a covalent bond with sulfur atom and displacing the hydrogen ion. This causes the enzyme to lose its ability to catalyze reactions.** Vaccines can have heavy metals such as, mercury; and almost all vaccines have aluminum (super conductor.)

It **is known that poisons and contaminants can adversely affect enzyme activity, abnormalizing it; vaccines' unnatural to human biology chemicals are abnormalizing!** Enzymes are bundles of amino acids. Science has discovered 50 amino acids however, only 20 amino acids are absolutely needed. It is crucial to have a normal biochemistry that produces the twenty amino acids needed to make proteins by humans to survive and be optimally healthy and, the required five nucleotides. Of the 20 amino acids, 9 are defined as essential in adults because an adult can synthesize the others 11 however, **children require them all.** If reaction controlling or magnetically stronger unnatural to human biology chemicals reactants are in the mix, bioreaction degeneration will result and Autism can be spawned. It would be extremely disturbing if snake venom were in vaccines and it is as, disturbing that **heavy metals, mercury derivative (thimerosal), aluminum or other unnatural to the body chemicals are in vaccines.** There is no controlling reason to have such, **chemical poisons** in children's vaccines! **If the EPA considers mercury toxic to the environment; CLASSIFY IT TOXIC TO HUMANS!** The chemicals that have been found in vaccines are not part of the cycles that create those biological compounds required for life in fact, the unnatural to human biology chemicals interfere with the cycles that create the needed for health biological compounds. There is no excuse to have such, abusive chemicals in vaccines and to mandate such, vaccine chemicalizations is to MANDATE MASS CHILD ABUSE BY VACCINE CHEMICALIZATION!

We have seen to it or allowed it to occur or are blind to the fact, that unnatural to human biology chemicals have infiltrated the water we drink, the food we eat, the air we breathe, our environment and the vaccines we inject. These chemicals are the stumbling blocks of health and the building blocks of disease and/or CHEMICALIZATION Autism. The water authority has been closing wells everywhere because they are polluted. We dump batteries and toxins in our landfills that leach poisons into the ground and our water supply and the food that we eat is grown in toxic dirt and watered with toxic content. We are all being chemically compromised and are much more susceptible to cancer and CHEMICALIZATION Autism for it. There are those politicians or leaders that despite the clear understanding that such, chemicalization causes cancer and Autism remain blind to it and there are everyday citizens or parents that choose to ignore the truth or be blind to it. The blind that lead the blind will both fall into a bottomless pit of unhealth and despair. The fact, that today's adults and children are chemically compromised is more reason to assure that babies, infants and small children are not further chemically compromised with vaccines that have unnatural to human biology chemicals. We want to freely be able to choose to be vaccinated and obtain the potential benefits from vaccines however, it must be a rational choice therefore, we desperately need as, consumers of healthcare; SAFER vaccines. Recognize that chemicalization by injection is by far the worst type or kind of exposure because it is unabated; its chemicals have full impact as, it circulates passing the blood brain barrier to dope the brain cells. This can set you FREE; no longer be blind, safeguard yourself and children from chemicalization!

The cycles that make the required for optimum health biological compounds rely upon enzymes and other proteins to move the atoms and molecules. Metabolism is the total of all the chemical reactions we need to survive; vaccine chemicals abnormalize metabolism as its alien to the body chemicals take part in reactions. Make a tree good and the fruit will be good, make a tree bad and the fruit will be bad. Make your children's biochemistry good and pure and their chemical reactions, enzymes, proteins and/or biological compounds will be good, making your children healthy; without **CHEMICALIZATION Autism**. It is true to a large degree that what you eat affects your health; it is true that what chemicals you inject to an exponentially higher degree affects your health. What the body manufacturers is totally dependent upon the chemicals within. Optimize your internalization of chemicals strategy and you optimize your health! Internalize unnatural to human biology chemicals by injecting those chemicals found in non-**SAFER** vaccines and you do not optimize health but instead, optimize the spawning **CHEMICALIZATION AUTISM**.

The body is like a factory, there are thousands of combinations of those twenty amino acids; they are used to make all the proteins in your body. Amino acids bond together to make long chains. Those long chains of amino acids are also called proteins. There are the Essential Amino Acids: Histidine, Isoleucine, Leucine, Lysine, Methionine, Phenylalanine, Threonine, Tryptophan, and Valine. There are the nonessential Amino Acids: Alanine, Asparagine, Aspartic Acid, Glutamic Acid. There are the conditional Amino Acids: Arginine (**essential in children**, not in adults), Cysteine, Glutamine, Glycine, Proline, Serine, and Tyrosine. Think about what can go wrong with the biological manufacturing of all the amino acids and its complicated long chains (proteins) when you inject a baby with unnatural to human biology chemicals which are alien reactants that have abnormal to the body chemical reactive propensity and disruptive to reaction magnetic fields. You do not need a study confirming that such, an occurrence causes abnormality; it is too obvious a conclusion. **A body with a divergent from normal biochemistry is divided against itself and who's health will be destroyed by it. Certainly, our children's bodies cannot escape the efficiency of the normal biochemical processes going on in each cell, so it is probable that children who are injected with vaccine's unnatural to human biology chemicals cannot escape its chemical influences or processes.**

Magnetic fields of unnatural to the human body chemicals found in vaccines resonate the cells and impact biological production within its zone of effect. Such, chemicals have traits that can adversely affect the outcome of bioreaction and its production! Human biology is an intricate and complex working of chemical reactions for production of what is required to be optimally healthy and/or not Autistic. Polar amino acids adjust themselves in a certain direction. Chemical traits allow amino acids to point towards water (hydrophilic) or away from water (hydrophobic). Growing chains of amino acids can twist and turn when they are being synthesized according to chemical traits and/or under its magnetic field of influence. The balance of biochemistry is very sensitive and altering it with unnatural to human biology chemicals is destructive to health and/or toward human biology and/or physiology and functionality. A study that needs to be done, if it is humanly possible, is to analyze the quantity and quality of the bio products such as, but not limited to, enzymes of a child proximate to being vaccinated and of those proximate to being diagnosed with Autism and compare to an unvaccinated healthy child. Bio productions such as, enzymes will be shown to be abnormalized by quantity and/or quality; enzyme control is lost. Immune cell production levels will be shown to be abnormal etc.

In order for one neuron cell to communicate or send an impulse to another neuron cell the synapse between the neurons must have proper chemical geometry and/or normal neurotransmitters need to be present. The presence of unnatural to the body elements have abnormal magnetic fields that can disrupt amino acid production. Putting science aside, the sheer logic of it is overwhelming; you cannot inject substances that you do not require for life and expect health perfection or not expect abnormality. Logic dictates that chemicals play a major role in Autism. Those unvaccinated are not benefiting from vaccination however, they are not being induced to suffer Autism. The Amish people and the Christian scientists who do not vaccinate hardly ever suffer Autism. Statistics, is food for logical deduction; what does your logic tell you? It is theorized that Autism is partially a protein disorder however, the protein disorder stems from biochemical disarray due to unnatural to the body chemicalization.

Even our (blood) hemoglobin is a mass complexity of amino acids. Unnatural to human biology chemicalization from vaccination explains why so many types of health problems are reported after vaccination. Even enzymes are proteins (a mass of amino acids). Enzymes are biological proteins that act as catalysts that help complex reactions occur in the body. Enzymes are everywhere in the body and we could not survive without them. Enzymes are very diversified and designed for specific tasks. Enzymes are very specific catalysts and usually work to complete one type of function. Certain enzymes have certain jobs; there are enzymes for intestine cells that are specific for protein digestion and another enzyme is specific for carbohydrate digestion, there are enzymes specific for neural cells, specific for saliva cells etc. **The complexity of problems of someone suffering with Autism indicates that the vaccine chemicalization is abnormalizing amino acid production and its combination. The alien to the body magnetic disruption and the abnormalizing chemical propensities of the vaccine chemicalization is causing children's building blocks of health (amino acids) to become stumbling blocks. Think before you allow such, injection; only consider SAFER vaccines!**

The main reason why vaccination is mandated is because it secures profits for **Big Pharma** and **Big Pharma lobbyists are making sure of it. Lobbyist are ruining America by hijacking government. As of 2018 there is an overwhelming 24,000 plus lobbyists and it is over a six (6) BILLION-dollar business. Big Pharma by itself has an outrageous task force of 13,000 lobbyists to push into regulation its self-serving unhealthy agenda and that is why more and more vaccines are mandated, that is why chemicals for profit remain in vaccines and that is why our children's best interest is not being best served and that is why parents must now step up to the plate of parenting in order, to protect their children from all these unamerican antics. Children's welfare is NOT best served under such, a one-sided power and purse of lobbyists. It has ruined our system of government; It is no longer government for the People and by the People instead it is bought and paid for regulation that keeps our innocent and vulnerable children under the oppression of vaccine chemicalization madness. Negative self-serving agenda has permeated every branch of government to the point of total control; our liberty is being destroyed and or safety being placed in danger because of it. We need SAFER vaccines that** can only be procured by a FREE and fair market place that is based upon freedom of medical choice!

Big Pharma and its cohorts of lobbyists have seen to it that mandated vaccination violate our Human Right to medical choice; all for the pursuit of unjustly unearned dollars. There is the fundamental Right to have control or self-govern over what can or cannot enter one's very own body. The concept of mandating the injection of whatever vaccines that Big Pharma's lobbyist manipulate into regulation is so wayward to this fundamental liberty that it should no longer be permitted in a freedom-based America. What healthcare to accept or deny for perfectly healthy children is strictly a parental decision and matter of utmost privacy. The unnatural to human chemicals for profit that continue to be in vaccines would not be there if we implement fully the TWO STEPS OF CORRECTION. Some incorrectly argue that the particles are so, small so, finite that it could not be harmful. With the advent of particles with a size inferior to 100 nm non-toxic materials become toxic and carcinogenic when sub-100 nm can become more toxic or carcinogenic. Perhaps, some toxic and carcinogenic materials become innocuous, but the opposite is usually true. For example, titanium was not known to cause health problems until the advent of titanium nanopowders. Vaccines will likely cause more problems with Nano-particles; not less. Parents should be FREE to refuse no matter what size the particles!

How much unnatural to the body chemicals can your baby internalize before the scale of bioreactions are tipped to abnormality? Irresponsibly those who are charged with protecting us have failed horribly to do so, they are hereby, the UNPROTECTORS for allowing bad chemicals to permeate our environment and be in children's vaccines. It was reported on 8/16/18 that Roundup Weed Killer found in Cheerios and Quaker Oats. Glyphosate is the active ingredient in Monsanto's Roundup weed killer, and at high levels, has been linked to cancer; parents must be concerned about what even small amounts are doing to their small children! Lucky Charms was also, found to have too high levels of this poison; how unlucky it is for those children who eat it! There are other foods that this toxin has permeated into and good old incredulous Monsanto's keeps driving its nasty product into our lives for profit. Interestingly, almost simultaneously with the above findings a jury, on 8/10/18, after a trial in a San Francisco Superior Court, returned a verdict in favor of Dewayne "Lee" Johnson, a former groundskeeper whose job required the use of Roundup and Ranger Pro weed killers. The jury rejected Monsanto's arguments that years of 'science' refuted Mr. Johnson's claimed link between Roundup and his terminal cancer diagnosis, (Case entitled: Johnson v. Monsanto Company, San Francisco Superior Court, case number: CGC016-550128). We need litigation liberty in vaccine cases!

Inequitably, parents claiming their children have been injured and/or been induced to be Autistic by vaccines that have toxic chemicals are forbidden to seek compensation or injunctive relief against Big Pharma (vaccine producers) because its lobbyist obtained an unconscionable liability shield that forbids it. Not having redress against Big Pharma is un-American and places Big Pharma above the law. Parents need to be conscious about chemical exposures and protect their children accordingly, do not leave it up to the UNPROTECTORS. How many chemicals will you allow to be injected into your babies highly susceptible systems until you start to refuse it? You can choose to allow your children to eat Roundup breakfast or refuse to let them eat it but, you must allow a vaccine chemiclization; YOU SHOULD BE FREE TO REFUSE ANY UNWANTED CHEMICALIZATION!

Parents need to be FREE to refuse what parents consider a vaccine that is too dangerous to inject; without legal restriction. Vaccination mandates divide parents from their children, severing and nullifying parents' liberty and legal ability to protect children from what parents deem a vaccine that is too dangerous to inject; it is a perversion of justice and renders America upside-down. You cannot strip away parent's authority, power and knowhow of doing what they think best for children and have safer children or a FREE America. One must be FREE to not allow their children to become drunk with unnatural to human biology chemicals; not permitting one's children's brain cells to be doped by injection with objectionable chemicals that could be or are in vaccines. You would be living in reality and be completely accurate and correct to state that unnatural to human biology chemicals are enemy number one to your children's optimum health or welfare. Bad chemicalization causes abnormal bioreactions, abnormality, malfunction, disease proliferation, cancer, abortion and yes, it causes CHEMICALIZATION AUTISM. I will end this chapter repeating the all-important words, VACCINATION WAS MADE FOR MAN, NOT MAN FOR VACCINATION! Do not be a statistic of DIAGNOSIS AUTISM.

There are negative to health consequences after being injected with unnatural to human biology vaccine chemicals that arise from the chemicals' reactive propensities. In addition, there are the negative to health consequences from the strong magnetic resonance of certain chemicals in vaccines as, it rages throughout the circulatory system and when it surrounds or enters cells. In the back of every parents' mind, when in the pediatricians' office, is the possibility of harm from the proposed vaccination. Some parents allow the injection because they do not want the responsibility of the decision and many are coerced into it even though they think it could be to some degree injurious. All children have a degree of anxiety when the doctor comes at them with a vaccination needle and most if not all, children who have any degree of understanding about the controversy or safety concerns over vaccines have high anxiety as they stick out their arm to be stabbed with possible injection pain or harm. The following paragraph is about the mind/body connection and health problems that occur from being injected against your will and/or when you think it can or will cause harm and/or increase the risk of Autism. If the vaccine is or is not dangerous has no relevance to injuries caused by a sure mindset.

Analyzing what mental problems and/or physical problems can occur when parents are enforced or coerced to vaccinate their children against their will or subject their children to it when they or their children are afraid of it or have it in their minds that it is injurious or harmful reveals that to suffer vaccination under such, circumstances can cause harm to that individual because of one's mindset, in what is a result of "NEGATIVE PLACEBO EFFECT"; everyone has heard of the placebo effect; this is what is called a "NEGATIVE PLACEBO EFFECT". The placebo effect is a two-way road; if you think that the action you take will have positive results then there will be a positive placebo effect that will cause positive results despite the level of effectiveness of the drug or action whereas, if you think the action you take is bad for you or that the vaccine will cause negative to health results then there will be a NEGATIVE PLACEBO EFFECT that produces negative to health results in addition, to whatever unhealthy chemicals are in the vaccine.

When parents are convinced that a vaccine has chemicals that cause health problems and/or if the child that is to be vaccinated is afraid or is witness to their parents fear or anxiety or senses it, then if that child is injected that child will likely suffer a NEGATIVE PLACEBO EFFECT. In addition, if actual anxiety is caused it is harm that has adverse effects upon hormones, adrenalin etc. To receive a vaccine chemicalization under these circumstances can only cause more probability of abnormality or harm and/or Autism. It is rational to fear vaccines that are not tested with double- or triple-blind studies as, all drugs are usually tested. Vaccines are rushed through the system and released upon the public. Being fearful when a vaccine is an unnatural to human biology chemicaliztion is totally rational; be extremely concerned and protect accordingly!

What is the surest or best way to prevent Autism? Should parents be enabled to stop or prevent their children from being exposed to chemicals that parents think are dangerous? Do you want vaccines not to have unnatural to human biology chemicals such as, the chemicals used as, preservatives in vaccines that give vaccines very long shelf-life? Do parents know what is best for their children or does government? I hope by reading this book that you answer all these questions with confidence and conviction to protect your children from unnatural to human biology chemiclization by injection abuse. The most important question that I hope you can answer with authority after reading this book is the following: Will having vaccines and the vaccination delivery system based upon the TWO STEPS OF CORRECTION achieve and/or assure SAFER vaccines? Know that SAFER vaccines will exponentially decrease the chances of chemiclization Autism! Be safe not sorry; consider only SAFER vaccines for your children!

The mission for SAFER vaccines is more centered upon science, law of chemistry and biology than the emotional outcries of those being injured by unsafe vaccines and that is why I have not put peoples personal experiences with being injured by a vaccination in this book so, that the reader's mind is not overinfluenced by it and rather, the reader judges upon logic, science and common sense. However, the documented injuries from vaccines that are happening too frequently, can give clearer perspective of the need for SAFER vaccines. The courts have awarded over a Billion dollars to the multitudes proven injured by vaccine chemicalization. Trust that your natural biochemistry gives you the best chance at optimum health and trust that to distort the chemistry with vaccine's unnatural to human biology chemicals causes abnormal reactions and that equals abnormality and/or (AUTISM).

It can be considered not just negligent to lace vaccines with unnatural to human biology chemicals but rather, gross negligence to do so. Knowledge involves the accumulation of facts and it cannot be said that vaccine producers have no knowledge of the fact, that they are putting unnatural to human biology chemicals in our children's vaccine supply. It is common knowledge that many of the chemicals found in vaccines such as, but not limited to mercury derivatives and aluminum are chemicals or chemical compounds that are not part of the normal biochemical reactions of the body and cause abnormal to human biology reactions. Wisdom is the ability to apply knowledge to achieve the best result. Vaccine producers have not shown wisdom to produce SAFER vaccines. Knowledge is understanding that a tomato is a fruit, not a vegetable. Wisdom is knowing not to put tomatoes in a fruit salad. Wisdom is knowing not to put unnatural to human biology chemicals in our children's vaccines. To protect your family from being chemically compromised or to be protected from deception, adhere to the wisdom of GOD Himself. It is not enough to have the wisdom the world or what science offers. Knowing what GOD wants is divine wisdom. Do you think GOD wants your baby to be injected with alien, unnatural to normal biochemistry, chemicalizations? Perfect a Religious Exemption to not violate your religion.

It is hard to trust in vaccines or in vaccine producers when they have uncaringly, unwisely and in many legal opinions negligently, put chemicals such as, but not limited to mercury and aluminum in our children's vaccines; it is inexcusable and makes one feel a fool for having blindly trusted that the pharmaceutical industry would do right by our children. For more and more religious people, the question of vaccination has become a matter for one's religion perhaps, because people's trust has been so, violated. People are realizing that they are far better off securing children's safety with the parental Right to decide what is best for their children or have recognized such, chemicalization is defiling children's body and blood against GOD's Law and is therefore, a violation of one's religion. People are concluding that they should put their trust in GOD and not in for profit vaccinations that have been proven to be unnatural to human biology chemicalizations! Religious Exemption has become a required step to religious liberty to not be vaccinated! Whether vaccination be a cerebral decision, or one based upon religious belief it is a decision that must be yours to make; and not be enforced upon you by government.

If the United States has sovereign power to control its boarders as to what enters it certainly, individuals have sovereign power over what enters their body or rather, what can or cannot be injected into their blood. People have an inalienable Right of control over themselves and what will run through their blood and body. Your body is your temple and your religion may dictate that you must control what enters your body and safe keep your sacred blood according to what you know GOD wills. It is unjust and a violation of the Constitution to question or judge your religion. Going through the indignity of obtaining a Religious Exemption is presently, a necessary evil to protect what is only yours to protect! In your religious liberty to protect your children as your religion dictates always take into consideration that chemicals dictate reactions; health is completely dependent upon proper reactions and the avoidance of abnormal reactions.

Parents need to know exactly what chemicals is in a vaccine that is being contemplated for injection and be completely FREE to refuse it either because they do not know what chemicals is in the vaccine or because they know what chemicals is in the vaccine and think it not in their child's best interest. To put this problem of not knowing what chemicals is in a vaccine in perspective, would you buy a bag of food to feed your children without knowing what is in it? Most – if not all – people would answer this loaded question with a resounding "NO!" Yes, it is rational to want your child to be protected from childhood disease but, to do so without knowing what chemicals is in a vaccine leaves your child to the vices of possible improper medical intervention. Parenting requires parents to be vigilant as to what chemicals their children are exposed to. To live under the tyranny of mandated or enforced vaccination so infringes or violate parenting that it can no longer be permitted and promoted runaway negligence on the part of vaccine production. Indeed, to secure the safety of children we must be FREE to be parents and in that perfected freedom protect our children from unwanted and/or unhealthy chemicalization. Thank GOD for Freedom of Religion being there to protect us from an unwanted vaccination, if it violates our religion however, people need to be secure in their Parental Right to protect children!

POSITIVE HEALTH MEASURES

I f you think the wrong things about objective evidence, you will not get things right and lose the opportunity to improve because of it. If you think the earth is flat, you lose the opportunities that come from knowing the earth is round. If you think that unnatural to human biology chemicals do not have detrimental impact upon the biochemical reactions of the body, you lose the possibility of SAFER vaccines. Make no mistake, the injection of unnatural to human biology chemicals into tiny babies, small infants and little children is unhealthy to those vaccinated with such, chemicalization; it is spawning abnormality. All the SIGNS and/or SYSMPTOMS after vaccination point to health destruction by chemicalization. The SIGNS and/or SYMPTOMS which, occur after a vaccination validates that unnatural to human biology chemicals cause abnormality; the adverse reactions are billboards saying, attention! Even the CDC's grossly limited list of vaccine's adverse reactions is a strong enough message that vaccines cause abnormal reactions and/or abnormality. ABNORMAL reactions equal ABNORMALITIES! The well-known SIGNS and SYMPTOMS from vaccination, along with the sheer magnitude parental observations of their children's health demise proximate to vaccination and the Laws of Chemistry connects the dots of causation and draws a line in the sands of health that is crossed by chemicalization; it clearly points to what is spawning the Autism epidemic. POSITIVE HEALTH MEASURES for the prevention and recovery of CHEMICALIZATION AUTISM starts with understanding that it is unnatural to human biology chemicals which, cause Autism!

The chemicals you internalize will influence and/or DOMINATE the bioreactions of the body and determine whether you are healthy or Autistic. Being chemically, conscious is most wise! The biological chemical environment in and around our cells control whether we are healthy or sick. The chemicals within our body either keep pathogens in check or create an environment for the viruses and bacteria to multiply out of control to spawn or cause disease. The number one health measure is to prevent being exposed to anti-health chemicals; preserving the normal/natural chemical geometry is the most positive health measure. Parents who do not want their children exposed to bad chemicals or be injected with unnatural to human biology chemicals found in vaccines that are not the SAFER vaccine variety, must insist or demand it! Do not let someone's callous disregard of your wanting to protect your children from chemical injections, deter you! Any repressive measures that curtail an individual's autonomy to self-govern, self-regulate or self-preserve one's very own internal welfare and/or healthcare must not be tolerated. Parents' must not be stripped of their fundamental Right of protecting their children. If parents think vaccine chemicals are too dangerous or not in their child's best health interest; no vaccination should be given, end of story. Children need to have their parents protect their chemical integrity and parents need to be FREE to protect their children's natural chemistry. You must be FREE to prevent chemicalizations and save your children from being chemically compromised. If anti-health chemicals penetrate children, it can cause CHEMICALIZATION AUTISM. Vaccine chemicals are unnatural and unhealthy to the body!

When injured by vaccine injections take affirmative measures to reverse the unnatural chemicalizations. Do seek damages against the Vaccine Producer that manufactured the harmful vaccines. Once an injury takes place it is a difficult and stressful life ahead for child and parents however, there can be tremendous improvement if you purify the chemistry. Parents are all but abandoned by government; left to fend for themselves in the maize of Autism complexity and solely foot the cost of Autism. Natural healthcare can be of benefit whereas; giving medicine that **infiltrates an already chemically compromised victim** with more unnatural CHEMICALS, in an attempt to fight off a problem that was initiated by CHEMICALS in the first place; is unwise. The Autistic' should not add insult to injury and/or inject or take oral unnatural to the body drug/vaccine chemicalizations. Drugs are big business and may not be in your best interest.

The pharmaceutical industry is bent on selling the public more drugs and tries to get more and more people on **lifetime prescriptions**. It is estimated that in the United States **1 out of 4 adults** over the age 45 are taking a statin drug (Lipitor, Crestor, etc.) and they will be **on them for life**. All drug chemicals cause ADVERSE side-effects and/or health AILMENTS. Doctors prescribe more drugs to combat the problems caused by the first drugs that were prescribed. Your body is really quite efficient and effective at preventing and recovering from illness on its own naturally; you have an amazing innate intelligence. Many people are becoming logic stricken and do not want to get on the drug/chemical ingesting merry-go-round or want to get off of it. The Autism epidemic is spawned from injecting the anti-health chemicals of vaccines; to add insult to injury, by adding even more unnatural to the body chemicals, into an already chemically compromised individual is NOT health logical! We have all kinds of freedoms however, the decision if a drug and/or vaccine will or will not be internalized is among your most important and essential of fundamental freedoms!

The proper functioning of the mind, maintenance of optimum functionality and to best recover from improper function is crucially dependent on having the right chemicals and/or vitamin and minerals. My research indicates to prevent mind malfunction, mental breakdown, confusion, delusion, dementia and/or Alzheimer's disease and Autism that proper levels of vitamin B1 and B12 are essential. A lack of either B1 (Thiamine) or B12 (Cyanocobalamin is a man-made form of vitamin B12) can help prevent Alzheimer's and Autism. If I were to be diagnosed with either I would take mega-dosages of B1 and B12. The medical field should have come this conclusion long ago, and commonly highly recommend it however, because natural remedies are not as profitable as the hardcore drugs sales it is suppressed. There should be a golden rule in place that natural remedies which have no or close to nonexistent adverse side-effects,

MUST be wisely utilized first or at least contemporaneously with any drug prescriptions which are always fraught with adverse side-effects! One thing that Autism or Alzheimer patients do not need is to be violated with unnatural to human biology CHEMICALIZATION.

Food sources of thiamine include beef, liver, dried milk, nuts, oats, oranges, pork, eggs, seeds, legumes, peas and yeast. Foods are also fortified with thiamine. Some foods that are often fortified with B1 are rice, pasta, breads, cereals and flour.

Food Sources of Vitamin B12

Food	Micrograms (mcg) per serving	Percent DV*
Clams, cooked, 3 ounces	84.1	1,402
Liver, beef, cooked, 3 ounces	70.7	1,178
Nutritional yeasts, fortified with 100% of the DV for vitamin B12, 1 serving	6.0	100
Trout, rainbow, wild, cooked, 3 ounces	5.4	90
Salmon, sockeye, cooked, 3 ounces	4.8	80
Trout, rainbow, farmed, cooked, 3 ounces	3.5	58
Tuna fish, light, canned in water, 3 ounces	2.5	42
Cheeseburger, double patty and bun, 1 sandwich	2.1	35
Haddock, cooked, 3 ounces	1.8	30
Breakfast cereals, fortified with 25% of the DV for vitamin B12, 1 serving	1.5	25
Beef, top sirloin, broiled, 3 ounces	1.4	23
Milk, low-fat, 1 cup	1.2	18
Yogurt, fruit, low-fat, 8 ounces	1.1	18
Cheese, Swiss, 1 ounce	0.9	15
Beef taco, 1 soft taco	0.9	15
Ham, cured, roasted, 3 ounces	0.6	10
Egg, whole, hard boiled, 1 large	0.6	10
Chicken, breast meat, roasted, 3 ounces	0.3	5

*DV = Daily Value. The U.S. Food and Drug Administration (FDA) developed DVs to help consumers compare the nutrient contents of products within the context of a total diet. The DV for vitamin B12 used for the values in the Table is 6.0 mcg for adults and children age 4 years and older. This DV, however, is changing to 2.4 mcg as the updated Nutrition and Supplement Facts labels are implemented. The updated labels and DVs must appear on food products and dietary supplements beginning in January 2020, but they can be used now. FDA does not require food labels to list vitamin B12 content unless a food has been fortified with this nutrient. Foods providing 20% or more of the DV are considered to be high sources of a nutrient, but foods providing lower percentages of the DV also contribute to a healthful diet.

All vitamin and mineral requirements need to be updated.

There are many health generating measures however, the prevention of further chemical exposure is most essential and the total avoidance of injecting chemically laced vaccines into the bloodstream is of extreme importance. For a child, that has already been chemically compromised by vaccine injection, swinging the internal chemical pendulum from unnatural and unhealthy into natural and healthy, arrests the chemical upheaval from vaccination chemicalization. Enrich the chemistry with vitamins and minerals and prevent further chemical abuse! Seek the advice of a physician in considering these essential to health measures but, do make sure that the health decisions are yours; not the doctors!

Here are some basic essentials to combat the chemicals that cause AUTISM and that RESTORE HEALTH. Eat organic super nutrition foods which are high in vitamins and minerals, the building blocks of health; be sure the food your Autistic child consumes is pesticide-free and fertilizer-free and not genetically mutated. Learn from (BEST IF ORGANIC.com or BEST IS ORGANIC.com) why organic is best. Read food packaging labels usually, the shorter the list of chemicals in your food the better. Eat only chemicals that are indigenous and harmonious with the body or what the body needs to build and maintain health. Do not over indulge or stress the body. Do not eat foods with dyes such as, yellow dye that is in Kraft's food company's macaroni and cheese products.

Steer completely clear from ingesting chemicals such as, azodicarbonamide, a chemical that makes bread spongy and is also, used in rubber-soled shoes and in the production of foamed plastics such as, gym mats. Realize how deceitful or deceptive and misleading it is to use azodicarbonamide and how the chemical industry's puppet government allows for the deceit; while placing all our lives at risk. The tell tail sign or best indicator that bread is spoiling is that it gets stale or hard; this tells us that it has lost its vitamins and minerals and is no longer healthy to eat. Azodicarbonamide makes bread forever spongy and thereby, the bread does not get hard or appear stale, not alerting you of its decay; the FDA allows this deception and harm. Check the ingredients before you eat anything. The drug/chemical industry lobbies for their unfettered insane ability to have their chemicals used and that vitamins and natural products are constantly, under attack.

Read ingredient labels, if the words of the ingredients are very long or the list of ingredients is very long; it usually indicates that you should not eat it. Do not eat foods processed or packaged in foreign countries like China, Korea or India, they could be tainted; the FDA knows that these countries do not have as good safety standards and yet it allows it. Do not eat foods with monosodium glutamate, also known as MSG or sodium glutamate; be aware that they keep changing its name to fool the consumer of its toxic existence, by misleadingly labeling MSG as yeast extract or hydrolyzed vegetable protein, HVP, stock broth, natural flavors or autolyzed protein. Be acutely aware of what chemicals have already been banned in Europe and why. Do not over-eat acidic food; eat alkaline or alkaline forming foods (drink Bragg's organic apple cider vinegar drinks). Check your acid/alkaline levels (pH), the blood's pH is best slightly alkaline, 7.4 or higher. The pH of saliva and urine will be more acidic than the blood because of proteins; you can check it with Litmus paper, keep it above 6.7 pH. The BODY HEALS BEST when slightly ALKALINE whereas, cancer and most diseases flourish in acidosis; chemicals and/or diet dictate ph.

Drink lots of clean water to help detoxify. For two weeks drink distilled water and then drink water which has no chlorine or harmful chemicals. Drink highly alkaline (9.5 pH) water and have no carbonated (CO_2) beverages. Avoid any and all mold. Increase loving contact, do not assault the senses, practice brain relaxation and rebooting, spend time meditating and absorbing nature's beauty. Have massages, correct spinal distortion, have acupuncture, meridian therapy and good nutrition. Regularly, expose your eyes and skin to a healthy degree of sunshine (but not while on drugs) and breathe clean, fresh air.

Make sure children's magnetic fields are not being manipulated or distorted. Prevent magnetic brain level interference by not placing the headboard of their beds adjacent to an electric outlet and absolutely not near the wall where the main power lines enter the house. Neurotransmitters at the neuron synapse can be caused what I call, "synapse arching unrest". Autistic children cannot rest when they supposed to and their exposure to electric and/or a significant electric magnetic field contributes to this. Chemical doping of brain cells from vaccine CHEMICALIZATIONS disrupt normal neuron synapse function.

Know that prescription drugs are chemicals that all have negative to health consequences when taken. Medication has its place, but do not overly, medicate or medicate unnecessarily or medicate if efficient and effective natural means of caring for the problem are available. Do not ingest fake foods or foods that have synthetics and/or are laced with chemicals that highjack your mind or takes it over. The general rule is the longer it takes to prepare and cook the food and the faster the food spoils; the healthier the food is for you. Avoid additives, artificial flavors, preservatives and aspartame. Stop ingesting plastics; drink out of glass containers. When papillae of the tongue inflame; you likely ate something toxic. Walk down a cereal aisle and read the contents of the cereals, you will be amazed at the garbage/chemicals that are in most cereals. Most importantly, think twice and then think again about injecting any more chemically laced vaccines. These are healthful or normalizing actions, precautions and alerts. The goal is to do everything in your power to promote health and steer clear of things that are anti-health.

What the body eliminates is an indication that we should avoid consuming it. Drinking carbonated beverages stresses the body. Our body's mitochondria produce CO2 as a WASTE PRODUCT of cellular respiration and we constantly, eliminate carbon dioxide as we breathe out; this tells us that it is an unwanted poison. This enlightens us that to purposely, consume carbonated beverages is unwise; it stresses and burdens the body and is opposite of what human physiology requires in order, to be healthy. Drinking carbonated beverages may spur on a belch that can help relieve gastric discomfort but that is as far as it goes health sense wise. When we ingest carbonated beverages, certain amounts of CO2 are absorbed into the bloodstream therefore; drinking carbonated beverages further taxes the elimination of the CO2 from the blood and/or body and this is not health logical. Just as it is unhealthy to consume other chemicals and/or materials that the body is constantly doing its best to eliminate such as, sweat or urine or fecal material; it is logical to consume carbonations is unhealthy. Based upon the body's need to rid itself of the aforementioned; do not consume flatulent beverages. The logic of the body must be understood and emulated in order, to best remain healthy or to best regain health.

Concentrate on getting rid of toxins and eliminating their sources. Perspiration is a primary method to rid the body of unwanted chemicals; sweat the toxins out. The body has vast intelligent know how, "innate intelligence". The body is intelligently designed to use the millions of pores in the skin as passages to remove toxins. I said as it was occurring, that all the heroes of 9/11 or anyone else that breathed in all the pulverized chemicals from the Twin Towers, chemically compromised their health; it's obvious, unnatural chemicalization is always anti-health. Anyone that has been chemically exposed especially, from vaccine injections need to rid their bodies of unnatural to the body chemicals! If unnatural to the body chemicals remain they will cause abnormality in the individual and can cause problems hereditarily. When the chemically exposed have children of their own the children will have a higher frequency of abnormalities. Be FREE to have NATURAL chemistry or select your own chemistry and/or health and/or healthcare.

We are made of water, chemicals and gas. Chemistry can dictate whether we are generating health or degenerating it; to best preserve optimum health, we must not manipulate or bastardize our normal, sensitive chemistry. Let this be a light bulb moment; your chemistry dictates whether you are healthy or unhealthy and your RIGHT TO BE HEALTHY AND IN CONTROL OF YOURSELF allows you to prevent unwanted chemical vaccine injection exposure. The connectivity of the human brain endows it with complexity and the chemicals within us dictate to what is communicated in this connectivity. By natural law and by common sense, you control whether an injection of vaccine CHEMICALS will or will not enter your sensitive system and only parents have this natural Right and obligation to decide what is best for children.

The public should be taught that by doing what is naturally good for health you are surrounding yourself with layers of protection from disease and/or health problems. By taking natural health measures and preventing chemical exposures you are building layers of protection, like the cumulative benefits of adding air bags, seat belts, fog lights, automatic braking system and other safety features in a fast-moving motor vehicle. You are building protection, surrounding yourself with things that protect you, and reduce your risk of injury or illness by doing what is naturally good for the body and steering clear of chemical anti-health agents. The chemicals that have been found in vaccines are anti-health agents. You must control your own health by being in control of what will or will not enter your body and/or bloodstream. To preserve health, do our utmost to keep internally clean; not inject chemicals that are not natural to the body. Be FREE to reject injections; be FREE to protect your children; Free to keep their blood biochemistry pure!

All prescription drugs are made of unnatural to the body chemicals that will further chemically damage the body when taken; so only take them if you absolutely must and/or if natural means to health are unavailable. Attempting to reduce the harm from a chemical exposure with more chemicals is inherently, problematic; it is best if an Autistic individual minimizes their problems by minimizing their chemical exposures and sets the course for healing. The harmful chemical exposure impact should be dealt with as soon as possible because the longer the body remains festering in a toxic exposed state, with no health normalizing and regenerating steps taken, the greater the chance of an acute condition becoming insidious or chronic and the greater possibility of Autism or permanent injury.

THE CHEMICALS THAT WE COME IN CLOSE CONTACT WITH OR THAT WE INJECT INTO OUR BLOODSTREAM DIRECTLY AND INDIRECTLY AFFECT US; ONE'S STATE OF HEALTH IS AFFECTED BY THE CHEMICALS THAT SURROUND AND PENETRATE OUR CELLS. You can maintain health and/or prevent Autism by governing and/or controlling what chemicals shall or shall not enter your body. Unhealthy chemicals must be avoided whereas; the right chemicals give you the right health results. Unlike vitamins and minerals that are required to stay healthy and repair the body; unnatural vaccine chemicals are destructive. Chemical infiltration begins degenerative to health processes that can be reversed however, there is a point of no return; when damage could be permanent. Time is of the essence when it comes to reducing chemicalization affects.

Autism prevention is a matter of maintaining the natural homeostatic chemistry and/or proper chemistry in order, to effectuate the complex biological functions. Recovery from Autism is a matter of correcting and/or naturalizing the chemistry in order, to re-establish biological function efficiency and effectiveness. Reset for an optimum chemical environment of health by developing life style and treatment regimentations, which promotes healing; this requires excluding unnatural chemicalizations. We must have the liberty to command our internal being and/or healthcare destiny; being FREE to decide what is best for one's welfare and control the healthcare of our children. Be enabled and/or empowered to follow one's own health decisions; this entails liberty to avoid chemical vaccine exposures, if one so desire. Moreover, you must have liberty to solely rely upon the type of healthcare you think best for your children or for yourself!

According to the World Health Organization (DATA and STATISTICS), "Proper environmental management is the key to avoiding a quarter of all preventable illness..." Maintaining internal chemistry is the key. Logically, maintaining the proper internal environment is even more important. Avoiding unnatural to the body vaccine chemicals entering the internal environment is essential to remaining healthy. The result of vaccine chemicals being injected into the susceptible bloodstream of children is that the vaccine chemicals manipulate or denaturalize the normal essential chemistry of the bloodstream. Chemical reactions and/or titration experiment in the lab give a glimpse into the chemical reactions within the human body; as they are all under the same universal laws of chemistry. When the natural blood chemicals are mingled or mixed with the injected vaccine chemicals the needed for health chemical reactions are disrupted and the chemical reactions reflect the presence of the vaccine chemicals. Maintaining the internal chemistry is important to prevent Autism and restoring it; stimulates Autism recovery.

If a titration experiment could be accomplished within the body, the universal truths of chemical interactions would affirm that altering the internal chemical homeostasis with unnatural to the body chemicals and/or alien chemicals to the normal bio-chemical reactions of the body; is distorts normal reactive results. Vaccine chemicals have negative impact upon homeostasis; the biochemical reactions and interactions necessary for optimum health. People must be FREE to refuse vaccine chemical disruption. Good parenting requires not exposing children to the present chemicals of vaccines; Vaccine Producers must be prompted to produce vaccines with no anti-health agents. Parents must see to it that children are offered safe vaccines, vaccines with no chemicals that are alien, unnatural to the body. The explosive Rate of Autism drives us to instill the TWO STEPS OF CORRECTION with laser-like focus. Perhaps, the TWO STEPS are the most important of the POSITIVE HEALTH MEASURES.

Universal chemical reactive principles and laws reveal that when alien, unnatural to the body or foreign to the body chemicals are added to the natural, inherent chemical mixture of the body, it causes chemical reactive chaos. The normal reactions of the body can no longer be expected, relied upon or taken for granted after a chemically laced vaccine injection insult. The chemical reactions in the body must adhere to these universal chemistry laws just like in the chemistry lab therefore; a change in the natural chemistry is a change from normal and the severe virulent chemicals found in vaccines take reactive abnormal control. **MAKE INFORMED DECISIONS AND CELEBRATE YOUR FREEDOM OF DECIDING WHAT IS BEST FOR YOUR CHILDREN! The present unhealthy state of chemically laced vaccines, the immoral mandate of enforcing unwanted vaccinations and the ridiculous unwise escape of Vaccine Producers from vaccine induced injury liability are the root of all evil that spawns Autism.**

The normal reactions that are needed to take place to remain healthy are chemically interfered with or altered by the presence of alien, foreign to the body chemicals. **A chemical entanglement occurs** between the unnatural to the body chemicals and the inherent natural chemicals of the body, this causes abnormality and/or **transformation into Autism.** The reaction of vaccine chemicals with the native chemicals of the body **disrupts the natural environment into reactions of transformations and/or mutations.** This creation of alien to the body reactions causes a gamut negative to health products, producing ill health and/or Autism. Keeping the body free of vaccine chemicals is a most **POSITIVE HEALTH MEASURE.**

The very presence of certain toxins in and around your cells can dictate to your cell's genes, abnormally, triggering your genes, commanding the wrong reactions to take place, stimulating deleterious abnormal responses. Injected vaccine chemicals eventually surround and/or enter your cells therefore, not only chemically altering the normal reactions that can cause a critical mass chemical syndrome but also, trigger genes to create abnormality; both cause Autism. Do not throw the chemical dice by injecting unnatural chemicals; the odds are against you, it is probable that health will degenerate, and Autism develops. Decrease the risk of Autism by cleaning-up vaccines and not exposing children to anti-health chemicals. Parents must be **FREE** to protect children from chemicalization.

UNNATURAL to the body chemicals can induce the nervous system to not relax when it is supposed to relax instead, the child is jumpy and/or hyperactive. Negative chain reactions and abnormal productions are brought on by the presence of these harmful chemicals. In this instance the synapses of our neurological system that are dependent upon the natural, specific and proper presence of neurotransmitters are falsely manipulated by these foreign to the body chemicals. Chemicals can alter the normal level of impulses traveling across neuronal synapses; they mimic or act as neurotransmitters, causing neurological chaos and/or unrest. These children abnormally cannot relax, even when they try or physiologically are supposed to; Autistic children often display this unrest. **Unnatural chemicals are the stumbling blocks of health and building blocks of neurological disconnect from the normal; relaxation and/or proper impulses are affected.**

Unfortunately, vaccinations are unwisely a one size fits all approach. Vaccine dosages are the same whether one is large or small, of one age or another, girl or boy, antibiotic dependent or super healthy, have a cold or a fever at time of vaccination; making the chemical exposure risk greater for some. Children with substantial less mass or are not as developed or already have drug chemicals in their delicate systems are more susceptible or at greater risk of **CHEMICALIZATION AUTISM. The one size fits all approach of vaccinations is not the practice of good medicine,** it falls way short of the realm of proper medicine, breaches the good standard of the practice of medicine and is **NOT** in the best interest of the child.

The rational parent would not want their children treated in this one size fits all fashion. Always, remain in control of your internal natural chemistry; do not set into motion any chemical disturbance. The slightest change in our internal chemistry can lead to alien abnormalities, which can be devastating to health. A change in the elemental composition of the blood and/or brain cellular chemistry can lead to a world of difference and end results. **You must be in control of your health destiny. Your children depend on your guidance; it is for you to decide if your children shall have vaccine chemistry. Keep the blood and/or brain chemistry PURE and you will be as healthy; this is a most POSITIVE HEALTH MEASURE!**

The practice of good medicine dictates that healthcare should be individualized, specifically, designed and geared for the needs of the individual; taking into account an individual's specific body type, weight, age, maturity level, health history and/or present health/sickness status. The proper and good practice of medicine require having the timing of the vaccination and the vaccination itself adjusted to consider patient specific needs and/or the patient's individual health status and/or body make-up. The vaccine proposed for injection must be specifically geared for the individual patient! It is common sense and is healthcare logical that vaccine quantity be adjusted to patient specifics.

Vaccinations should be of a different quantity and potency and/or antigen level to meet the specifications of the individual's needs thereby, be suited for the individual patient and vaccines must be prompted to have NO anti-health propensities and/or unnatural to the body chemicals. Vaccinations must become much more personalized and/or individualized to prevent or decrease vaccine induced injuries. It is the bad practice of medicine to treat individuals generally and/or merely with a herd mentality. The mandated vaccination law treats people like herds of cattle and/or sheep people; branding an **ENSLAVED** public with vaccinations. Vaccination compliance scars or illness or side-effects are commanded to be endured by our children. **Wrongfully, it is required that we produce proof of vaccination in order, to enter school; we must prove that our children are vaccination compliant SLAVES.**

Currently, modern healthcare has it as, improper to treat patients in an inhumane way or **like sheep people; that have no individuality, or personal say in their very own healthcare**. Sometimes, at a court house, people are made to go through the indignity of being lined up, on long vaccination herding lines to submit their children for a coerced and/or enforced vaccination. These **human cattle lines** vaccinate the masses without a good standard of medical practice; there is no good standard requirement of health history or asking of health status and no health examination. **The erroneous vaccination laws treat our children and their parents with indecency and as if we have no individuality and Right to the quite enjoyment of our own lives and healthcare. Humane, voluntary healthcare is a POSITIVE HEALTH MEASURE! Keeping your biochemistry pure is a health priority!**

Health factors should be taken into consideration to **tweak dosages** to be much more specific for the individual's makeup and/or needs in order, to **vaccinate with less risk of injury**. It would be very wise not to vaccinate a child at the time that the child has a fever, is on antibiotics or shows signs and/or symptoms that indicate the child is more at risk of injury from vaccination. Honest studies need to be performed to determine when it is the optimum time to vaccinate or more importantly, **when it is time not to vaccinate**. Every chemical in vaccines should be studied for their impact upon health. There have been minimal studies performed on how the presence of chemicals in vaccines could cause health problems. Know what chemicals are in vaccines and protect your children accordingly.

With the prevalence of Autism always on the rise, at epidemic level, this no time to stick your research head in the ground, **know the risks; make intelligent, informed decisions**. Information is power, to know what is in vaccines, becoming armed with the knowledge of vaccine chemical propensities; is information power that is vital and a **POSITIVE HEALTH MEASURE**! The Autism epidemic commands you be more cautious, not less and that unbiased research be done and/ or without conflicts of interest. An honest, unbiased research scientist is a humble person, aware of what his study does or does not show and/ or what his study does not know but, continues nevertheless to seek answers. **PARENTS NEED ABSOLUTE CONTROL OVER THE PREVENTION OF CHEMICAL EXPOSURE ESPECIALLY, THE VACCINATION KIND!**

This is about parents protecting their children from unwanted, perceived of too dangerous to inject chemicalization. You can mask the real issue by postulating that children have a Right to be protected from childhood disease and/or Right of decision about how to protect oneself from childhood disease however; parent's Right of deciding for their children is controlling and/or parental protection of children from chemicalization harm supersedes. The law cannot pigheadedly ASSume to know babies', infants' and children's decisions about vaccination and/or how they would prevent childhood disease; the law cannot be based upon mere conjecture. Parents have always been their children's voice and/or protectors; parents do for their children what they cannot do for themselves and are vested with making children's life decisions, until children are no longer children and are of age and maturity to make informed health decisions.

In general, parents' hold children's best interest! It is traditional for parents to determine what is in their children's best interest; the determination of whether vaccines are safe and/or the decision to vaccinate or not, must be decided by none other than, the children's parents. Parents are not always perfect decision makers but, they have no conflict of interest in determining whether a vaccine is safe or unsafe for their children and/or if it is in children's best interest! Whereas, vaccination is far from perfect, in that they are CHEMICALIZATIONS and all have adverse side-effects and the mandated vaccination system is fraught with conflicts of interest, when it comes to determining if vaccination is or is not safe and/or is in the best interest of children. In addition, religious belief also, supersedes the mandate. Your body is your temple; parents must be FREE to have religious beliefs about health! PARENTAL DECISION CONTROL OVER VACCINATION IS A POSITIVE HEALTH MEASURE!

Every foreign to the body chemical that has been found in vaccines must be told to the potential vaccination recipient and each and every unnatural to the body chemical **MUST BE THOUROUGHLY STUDIED FOR ITS NEGATIVE TO HEALTH PROPENSITY**. Each chemical's individual affects, their interactive affects and their accumulative affects must become known and given to the public. Their effects on an individual's health who is overweight, diabetic, large mass compare to small mass, one age of development or maturity compared to another, anti-biotic dependent or not and highly allergic or not need to be understood. Why all kinds of negative side-effects are caused after vaccinations or why health problems like irritable bowel syndrome is caused by vaccinations must thoroughly be researched. **Perhaps, the greatest POSITIVE HEALTH MEASURE is for parents to be informed and to be in control of their children's vaccination destiny!** Postponing all these vaccinations until a greater immune system maturity occurs may be safer and is another important, **POSITIVE HEALTH MEASURE**; parents must be **FREE** to allow children's immune system to come on line; become more mature before injecting.

Parents have a basic instinct to protect their children and children are best off under this innate intelligence. Parents must enjoy the blessings of protecting their children from any conceived of harm and in the instant case; the conceived of vaccination harm and/or chemicalization. To deny parents their Right to Self-determine healthcare is an egregious injustice and not in children's best interest. Parents must be enabled to deny suspect or too dangerous to be inject vaccines. By GOD given law, parents' have the authoritative decision control and/or are the gatekeepers of their children's vaccinations; man-made law must be consistent with this. Refusing unwanted vaccines stimulates vaccine quality and/or safety. Liberty to control one's chemistry or homeostasis is essential to health and breeds purification of vaccines; protecting children. Be enabled to refuse chemical injections that you think too dangerous and you best protect children! No parent should be made to risk their children being chemically compromised or be forced to endure wondering if their children will be unscathed from vaccine chemicalization.

SAFER vaccines are a **POSITIVE HEALTH MEASURE** and all-important to patient confidence in vaccinations is the **SAFETY** of vaccines! The trust that the potential vaccination recipient places in the vaccinations is crucial to having a successful vaccination program. The great **TRUST BUSTER** is that vaccinations cannot be refused by parents; the legal mandate enforces vaccinations. No other medical intervention prevents good intentioned parents from refusing any proposed medical intervention for their children. **Trust is a key component to a patient's acceptance or denial of the intervention.** Trust in vaccinations is paramount to the mental and physical health of the individual. Waging lawsuits against Producers of harmful vaccines instills vaccine quality control and/or **SAFER** vaccines. **Without these above stimulators and assurers of vaccine quality; vaccine safety diminishes. Vaccine quality and/or safety entropy sets in and Vaccine Producers will stop caring about the outcome.**

A GIANT HEALTH STEP IS TO ASSURE NO ANTI-HEALTH CHEMICALS ARE IN VACCINES. Having no true informed consent/**DENIAL** requirement in order, for a vaccination to take place is an absolute **TRUST BUSTER; it automatically makes**

the vaccination suspect, gives a person pause and puts up a BIG red flag and light not to be vaccinated. Vaccine Producers hiding behind a rock of liability protection, shielding their company from just litigation is a **TRUST BUSTER; leaving vaccine production negligence unchecked and/or unwanted chemicals in vaccines.** It makes parents very suspicious of vaccination and gives good reason not to vaccinate. Parents reasonably, think that something underhanded is going on if they cannot refuse a vaccination or litigate against the Vaccine Producers if their child is injured by a vaccine. More and more parents have become educated about vaccines. Parents are no longer automatically or on the blind, agreeing to give their children a vaccine dosage instead, parents first obtain a good dose of intelligence about the vaccine, to learn if chemical dangers exist in the vaccine. Parents are regaining protective power over the welfare of their children!

If bad chemicals are not injected, children have a much better chance to be healthy and not Autistic. Injecting vaccine chemicals render the reactions of the bloodstream unstable. Vaccine chemicals throw off the normal course of reactions, expanding or contracting reactions and producing abnormal reactions and/or renegade production; the large-scale normal reactions become impossible. Children not exposed to vaccine chemicals have less infections, colds, otitis media and tonsillitis. Back in 1994, prior to major suppression of anti-vaccination information, Dr. Michael Odent, wrote in JAMA, there was a five times higher rate of asthma in pertussis immunized children compared to non-immunized. Parents need to be educated about the dangers of unhealthy chemicals. The controlling force of chemicals and/or their deleterious propensity must be yours to accept or deny; do not be dictated to inject harmful chemicals by government!

It is an imperative to optimum health to keep your baby's body, blood and especially, the developing brain, free of toxins or alien to the normal physiology or unnatural to human biology chemicals. GET THE BAD CHEMICALS OUT of vaccines, is a primary mission of the charity SAFER Vaccines; we, are all about SAFER vaccines for children. Injected vaccine chemicals circulate directly to the brain cells there is no built-in defense or filtering out of the chemicals; the chemicals are a direct hit. If you ingest poisons, the body's digestive/elimination system will not absorb the bad chemicals; the body attempts to rid what it does not need, eliminating the bad chemicals. Health is dependent upon proper chemistry. Synthetic food additives, Tran Fatty Acids, preservatives, pesticides, heavy metals and aspartame are harmful chemicals. Latex from the stoppers of vaccine vials and vaccine chemicals disrupt the normal chemistry. Brain function is dependent upon a normal health promoting chemistry. Vaccination exposed brain cells can malfunction. Parents must be free to protect the chemistry of children.

In deciding upon what health measures are best always remember, chemicals dictate reactions; health is completely dependent upon proper reactions and the avoidance of abnormal reactions. We must be FREE to decide what chemicals are best for ourselves and our children without government intrusion. We must be FREE to protect our children to the best of our ability. We must be FREE to live under the higher law of GOD and thereby, obtain a Religious Exemption from vaccine chemicalization. When it comes to vaccination there must be liberty of cognitive refusal and refusal on religious grounds! Be FREE to reject injections! Be FREE to follow your religious belief and/or become religious about health at any time; even if spontaneous in life.

Think about your child's biochemistry and how important it is to a babies' quickly developing biosystems! If you as a parent, keep your child's biochemistry normal, pure and/or unadulterated by unnatural to human biology chemicals; you have done the best health service for your child and have exponentially aided in your child being optimally healthy and not afflicted with Autism. Do make sure your child has all the chemical or chemical compounds that are the building blocks of health and do safeguard your child from being infiltrated with unnatural to human biology chemicalizations. Some people ask GOD what He would do in the matter of vaccination; would GOD want His children to be injected with any degree of chemicals that upset the natural and normal biochemical reactions of the body? Perhaps, GOD might approve of vaccination if the vaccine is a SAFER vaccine but, that is for YOUR religious belief to decide upon.

THANK YOU FOR TAKING TIME OUT OF YOUR PERTINENT TIME TABLE TO READ MY BOOK. I HOPE YOU STRIVE TO KEEP YOUR CHILDREN HEALTHY BY ONLY CONSIDERING SAFER VACCINES THAT DO NOT SO, CHEMICALLY COMPROMISE THEIR HEALTH.

Stand strong against what violates your religious belief, always be secure in the FREE Exercise of Religion. If vaccine chemicalization violates your religion, then do Perfect a Religious Exemption and by doing so, Secure Freedom of Religion. Stop chemically compromising children and there will be no chemically induced health problems!

Dr. Robert Caires, Esq., became inactive in practice to be very active in the mission to achieve much SAFER vaccines that do not so, readily chemically compromise children; for SAFER vaccines means safer children. Dr. Robert Caires has founded the charity SAFER Vaccines and vows to give all profit from this book into the charity. Have a blessed life, one that is not chemically compromised; may you and your family have the wisdom to be optimally healthy.

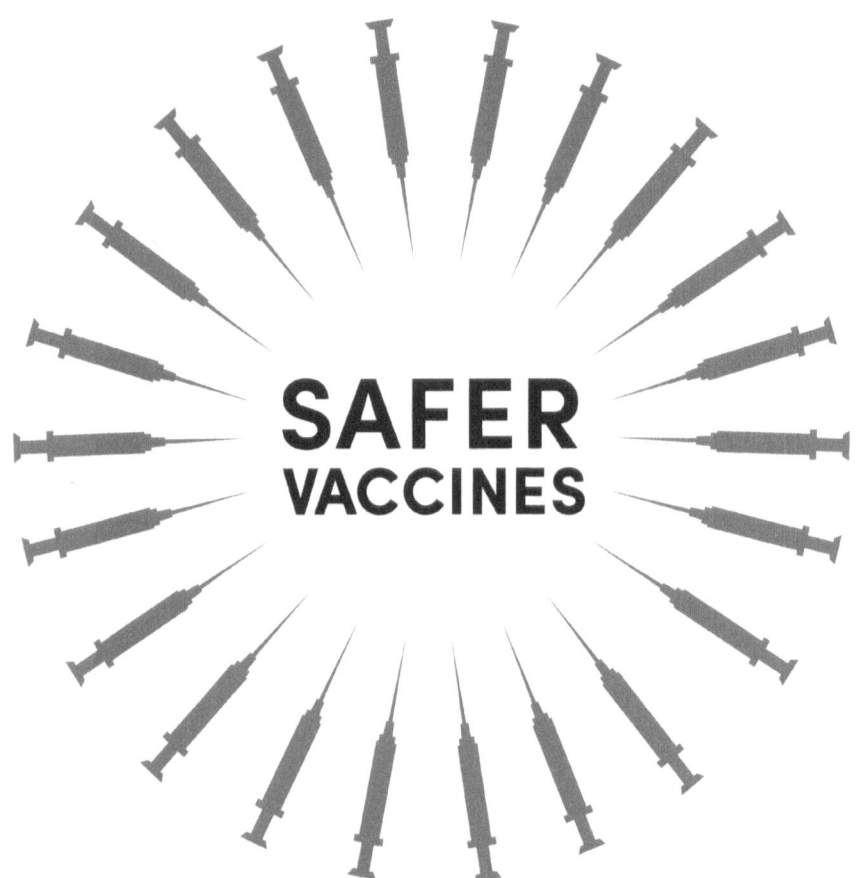

www.ingramcontent.com/pod-product-compliance
Lightning Source LLC
Chambersburg PA
CBHW030746180526
45163CB00003B/928